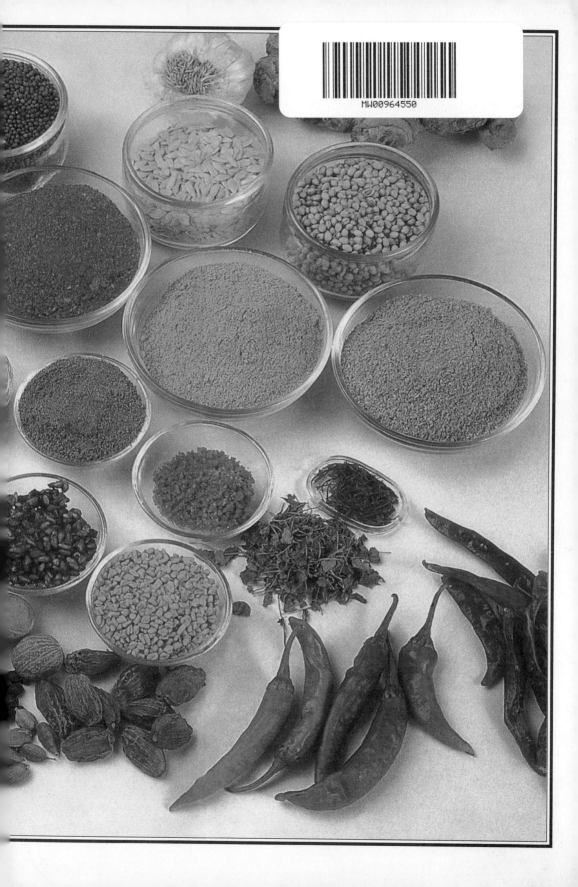

MW00964550

Dadi Maa

ke Nuskhon ka Khazana

Healing through Indian Herbs and Spices

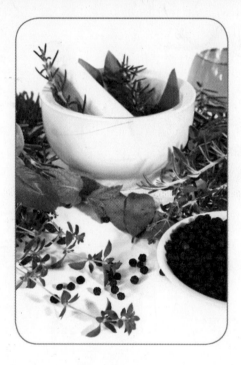

Nita Mehta

B.Sc. (Home Science), M.Sc. (Food and Nutrition) Gold Medalist

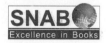

SNAB
Excellence in Books

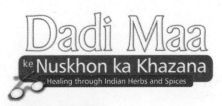

Dadi Maa
ke Nuskhon ka Khazana
Healing through Indian Herbs and Spices

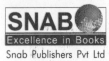

Snab Publishers Pvt Ltd

Corporate Office
3A/3, Asaf Ali Road, New Delhi 110 002
Phone: +91 11 2325 2948, 2325 0091
Telefax: +91 11 2325 0091
E-mail: nitamehta@nitamehta.com
Website: www.nitamehta.com

Editorial and Marketing office
E-159, Greater Kailash II, New Delhi 110 048

Food Styling and Photography by Snab
Typesetting by National Information Technology Academy
3A/3, Asaf Ali Road, New Delhi 110 002

Recipe Development & Testing:
Nita Mehta Foods - R & D Centre
3A/3, Asaf Ali Road, New Delhi - 110002
E-143, Amar Colony, Lajpat Nagar-IV, New Delhi - 110024

Distributed by :
NITA MEHTA BOOKS
3A/3, Asaf Ali Road, New Delhi - 02

Distribution Centre :
D16/1, Okhla Industrial Area, Phase-I,
New Delhi - 110020
Tel.: 26813199, 26813200
E-mail: nitamehta.mehta@gmail.com

Printed in India by Aegean Offset Printers, Greater Noida

Price: Rs. 245/-

"Not the Doctor, but Nature Heals."

From ancient times our grand mothers have treated us with their home remedies. Herbal remedies are the oldest and the most natural form of therapy. They heal gently with no side effects and most of them can be put together with common ingredients found in our kitchen.

This comprehensive book, will be useful for every person, who believes in the goodness of foods and herbs. Besides the remedies of various illnesses, also included are common symptoms of some problems, so that you could diagnose the problem before it turns too severe. The extensive index at the back of the book allows quick location of the remedies for your problem. Individual results from the use of remedies, may vary. Out of the remedies given under a particular problem, see what suits you and try one at a time only. First start with one remedy and follow it for a few days if it suits you, continue till the problem disappears completely. Repeat it once or twice a week for some more time.

Have complete faith and trust in the treatment and in God. Never follow any remedy half heartedly. Faith gives rise to hope and a positive approach always makes you attain your goal.

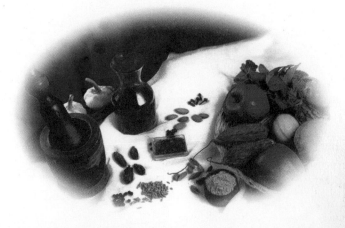

CONTENTS

ACIDITY

What is acidity?

❑ As a part of human body functioning, during digestion, the stomach secretes acid that aids in the breakdown of food. But when the gastric glands of the stomach produce excessive amounts of such acids, it leads to an ailment known as acidity.

Causes...

❑ Wrong diets, spicy foods, some medicines, consumption of alcohol.

Symptoms...

Acidity manifests, usually, after meals, while sleeping at night, or when one exerts pressure on the intra-abdominal area.

• Stomach pain, burning, bloating, burping, vomitting and nausea.

• Heartburn

• Formation of ulcers

Remedy (Nuskhe)...

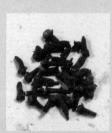

❑ Chew 1 clove *(laung)* after lunch and dinner.

❑ Chew a piece of black harad and an equal quantity of jaggery *(gur)* together. Drink a glass of water after that.

❑ To get relief from stomach ache due to acidity, grind ½-1 teaspoon fenugreek seeds *(methi daana)* with a little water to a paste. Add this paste to a glass of buttermilk *(lassi)* and drink.

❑ Drink coconut water 3-4 times a day. Drink a glass of coconut water every few (2-3) hours for a few days in case of very severe acidity.

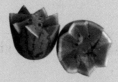

- Have a plateful of watermelon (*tarbooz*) and/or cucumber (*kheera*) every hour.

- Grapefruit like all other citrus fruits has an alkaline reaction in our bodies. Hence consumption of the fresh fruit or its juice is beneficial.

- Milk in combination with mangoes in the form of milk shakes, puddings or mango custard is called the ideal combination as the presence of milk supplies the protein, not present in the mango, that controls acidity.

- A glass of very cold milk with or without sugar is also very helpful.

ACNE

What is acne?

The sebaceous glands produce oil (sebum) which normally travels via hair follicles to the skin surface. When skin cells block the oil, follicles become plugged and bacteria begins to grow inside the follicles, causing acne pimples and cysts. In severe cases acne can involve the face, neck, back and scalp too.

Causes...

Hormonal changes that take place during puberty, secretion of excessive oil in the skin, pregnancy, menstrual periods, high stress levels, contraceptive pills, hereditary factors.

Symptoms...

There are two main types of acne: non-inflammatory and inflammatory.

Non-inflammatory acne: whiteheads and blackheads on the face.

Inflammatory acne: the whiteheads become inflamed and develop into red pimples.

Remedy (Nuskhe)...

❏ Never squeeze acne pimples because they spread more on doing so. Never let yourself get constipated. Avoid fried and spicy food.

❏ Clean face with cotton wool dipped in rose water 2-3 times a day. Do not use soap.

❏ Orange peel is very good in the treatment of acne. Grind the peel with some water to a paste and apply on affected parts. When oranges are not in season, dry peels in shade. Grind finely to a powder & store in an airtight jar. Mix with water & use.

❏ Mix 1 teaspoon lemon juice in 1 teaspoon finely ground cinnamon (*dalchini*) powder and apply on affected areas frequently. Sift the cinnamon (*dalchini*) powder to make it into a very fine powder.

❏ Crush a few garlic (*lasan*) flakes and apply on the face, once or twice a day. Swallowing 1-2 flakes of raw garlic regularly, helps further.

❏ Grind some *neem* leaves with water to a fine paste. Apply on infected area.

❏ Make a paste of ½ teaspoon each of sandalwood and turmeric (*haldi*) powder in a little water and apply.

❏ Grind some black cumin seeds (*shah jeera*) with a little vinegar (*sirka*) to a smooth paste. Apply on affected parts.

❏ Mix 1 teaspoon of lemon juice and 1 teaspoon of rose water (*gulab jal*). Apply on the face with a piece of cotton wool or face brush. Wash after ½ hour with plain water. Do it for 10-15 days.

❏ Dip a nutmeg (*jaiphal*) in unboiled cows milk *(kachcha doodh)* and rub on a stone *(sil)*. Apply on the face and let it dry. After it dries, rub gently to remove it. Wash off with warm water. Repeat twice a day for 3-4 days. You may also apply this paste at night before going to bed and wash the next day.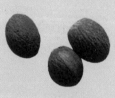

❏ Rub the bark of a neem tree from the inner side with a little water (like you do with a chandan stick). Apply the paste on the face and leave for ½ hour. Wash off.

ANAEMIA

What is anaemia?

Anaemia is a health ailment that takes place as a result of lack of red blood cells or haemoglobin in the body. Haemoglobin is a protein in your red blood cells that carries oxygen from your lungs to the rest of your body.

Causes...

Deficiency of iron in the body, lack of ability on the part of body to produce red blood cells, bleeding, menstruation, pregnancy, lactation, haemolysis (destruction of red blood cells), piles, hiatus hernia, peptic ulcer.

Symptoms...

A few anaemia symptoms include general weakness, dizziness and unconsciousness, headaches, fatigue, rapid heartbeats, shortness of breath and brittle nails.

Remedy (Nuskhe)...

❑ Have a ripe banana with 1 tablespoon honey everyday.

❑ Avoid drinking tea and coffee immediately after meals as the tannin present in these interferes in the absorption of iron from food.

❑ Juice of beetroot taken 1-2 times daily is an excellent remedy for anaemia, especially for children and teenagers. You may combine apple and beetroot for the juice.

❑ Mix 1 tablespoon amla juice with a ripe mashed banana and eat 2-3 times a day.

❑ Soak 8-10 almonds (*badaam*) and 1 teaspoon rice overnight. Remove outer skin of almonds and grind to a fine paste. Boil with 1½ cups of milk and a pinch of turmeric powder (*haldi*). Sweeten with sugar and drink for a few days, once a day.

- Soak 10-12 munakkas in water overnight. In the morning remove seeds and eat. Do this for 2-3 weeks.

- Drink juice of 125 gm spinach everyday, for 2-3 weeks.

- Almonds contain copper, which along with iron and vitamins acts as a catalyst in the synthesis of blood haemoglobin. Hence consumption of almonds is a sure shot remedy for anaemia.

- Although the iron content in grapes is very little it is very easily absorbed by the human body. Research confirms that having 300 ml of grape juice daily can be very beneficial in cases of anaemia.

- Pomegranate juice is very beneficial for anaemia and improves the quality of blood. Add some powdered cinnamon (*dalchini*) and cloves (*laung*) to the juice, or cinnamon (*dalchini*) powder and honey.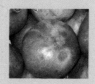

- The seeds of watermelon are high in iron. Eating dried and peeled seeds will be highly effective for people suffering from anaemia.

- Foods rich in iron are — honey, almonds, bananas, apricots (*khurmani*), raisins (*kishmish*), fenugreek (*methi*) leaves, fenugreek seeds (*methi daana*), lettuce or salad leaves, onions, spinach (*paalak*), grapes, tomatoes, carrots, gooseberry (*amla*), beetroots (*chukander*), apples, pomegranate (*anaar*). Have plenty of them if you are anaemic.

ANGINA PECTORIS

What is Angina pectoris?

Angina pectoris is chest pain caused due to insufficient blood and oxygen supply to the heart. It usually lasts for a few minutes, and an attack is usually relieved by rest or medicines.

Causes...

Angina is usually caused by exertion or emotional stress.

Symptoms...

Chest discomfort, heaviness, squeezing, burning or choking sensations. Apart from chest discomfort, anginal pains may also be experienced in the epigastrium (upper central abdomen), back, neck, jaw or shoulders.

Remedy (Nuskhe)...

❑ Mix well 2 teaspoons almond oil with 1 teaspoon rose oil. Rub gently on the chest, morning and evening.

❑ Boil 1 teaspoon fenugreek seeds (*methi dana*) in 1½ cups water. Strain and add 2 teaspoons honey. Take twice daily.

ANKLE - SWELLING & PAIN

What causes ankle swelling?

There are a number of possible causes for a swollen ankle. A) overuse that can lead to excess fluid accumulation and swelling. B) inflammation of the tendons. C) water- retention. D) certain medicines.

Remedy (Nuskhe)...

❑ Mix equal quantities of castor oil and lemon juice. Massage the affected area with this mixture. Also drink 1 cup warm water mixed with lemon juice and honey.

APPETITE LOSS (Anorexia)

What causes appetite loss?

Almost any infection can cause a loss of appetite. Sometime obesity that leads to diet fads that cause eating disorder; emotionally blocking the mind from eating.

Remedy (Nuskhe)...

❑ Mix half teaspoon each of—carom seeds (*ajwain*), fennel seeds (*saunf*), dried ginger powder (*saunth*), salt and black cumin seeds (*shah jeera*). Swallow about 3/4 teaspoon of this mixture with water—2-3 times a day.

❑ Take 2 teaspoons of amla juice and mix it with 2 teaspoons honey and 2 teaspoons lemon juice. Add 1 cup water and drink on an empty stomach every morning. To take out juice from fresh amla, remove seeds and grind the pulp into a fine paste. Tie it in a muslin cloth and squeeze out the juice. Whenever fresh fruits are not available, dried amla can be used. Soak 1 tablespoon of dried amla at night in a cup of water. Strain it the next morning. Add 1/8 teaspoon black pepper powder (*kali mirch*) and 2 teaspoon lemon juice.

Dilute it if necessary with water and drink every morning regularly on an empty stomach.

- ❑ Take ½ teaspoon black pepper powder (*kali mirch*) and 1 tablespoon jaggery powder *(shakkar)* mixed together.

- ❑ Cut 1" piece ginger (*adrak*) into small pieces. Add 1½ cups of water. Boil. Simmer for 2-3 minutes. Add milk and sugar to taste, and take it frequently like tea.

- ❑ The consumption of plums increases appetite and helps in the digestion of food.

ARTHRITIS

What is Arthritis?

Arthritis means inflammation (swelling) and pain in the bone and muscle joints.

Causes...

Lack of planned physical exercise can lead to softening of bones in old age. A supple body which is regularly exercised has few chances of developing arthritic complaints, unless the reasons spring from different sources. Overweight or obesity exerts unhealthy pressures on the bone joints — the weight-bearing zones of the body — which causes the bones to lose shape, leading to painful joint movements while bending, crossing knees, raising a hand, sitting down and so on. A golden rule to be followed religiously with all types of treatments for joint pains is to exercise the affected joint every day. Exercise goes a long way in helping movement, mobility of the joint and also in reducing pain.

Symptoms...

Nagging joint pains, swelling of joints, unexplained loss of weight, fatigue, deformity of joints.

Remedy (Nuskhe)...

❑ Squeeze half a lime/lemon in one glass of hot water (as hot as you can drink) and drink it. Have this 8-10 times a day. Having lemon juice might seem like a contradiction to what you have always believed that sour things are bad for joint pains but the action of lemon in the body is alkaline and its rich vitamin C content is valuable in the treatment of joint pains. I have personally benefited from this. Initially for a few days you might feel that the pain is increasing but gradually it decreases.

❑ A diet of only bananas for 3-4 days is advised. You can have 8-9 bananas a day.

❑ Make tea from papaya seeds and have 6-7 cups a day for at least 2 weeks.

❑ Have 1-2 garlic (*lasan*) cloves or 1 single pod garlic (*ek pothi lasan*), first thing in the morning.

❑ Mix 1 teaspoon of dry amla powder with 2 teaspoons of jaggery (*gur*) and have it twice daily for a month.

❑ Regularly massage affected joints with neem oil.

❑ Take a handful of fresh neem leaves. Grind them in the mixer with a little water. Strain. Add lemon juice and drink 1-2 times a day on an empty stomach (people prone to acidity avoid).

❑ Take equal quantities of asparagus seeds (*shatavari*), black cumin seeds (*shah jeera*), fenugreek (*methi daana*) seeds and carom seeds (*ajwain*). Powder and take ½ teaspoon every morning.

❑ Combine 6 teaspoons each of ginger (*adrak*) and caraway seeds along with 3 teaspoons of black peppercorns (*sabut kali mirch*) and grind into a fine powder. Have ½ teaspoon with water twice daily.

❑ Soak 1-2 teaspoons fenugreek seeds (*methi daana*) in a cup of curd or water overnight. Have it in the morning on an empty stomach.

❑ Grind fenugreek seeds *(methi daana)* to a fine powder. Swallow 1 teaspoon of it with water in the morning.

❑ Have 1 tablespoon juice of bathua leaves without adding any sugar or salt everyday, early morning on an empty stomach or at 4 pm in the evening, for 15 days . Do not eat anything 2 hours before or after taking it.

- On an empty stomach have 3-4 walnuts (*akhrot*) or fresh coconut for a few days.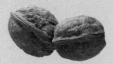

- Water treatment is considered to be very effective. The patient is asked to immerse the affected parts first in hot water for 3 minutes and then immediately in cold water for 1 minute. Hot water has pain-relieving properties, while cold water has curative properties. The two in combination help to remove the root cause of the pain.

- Mud pack on the aching joints, preferably the mud found on river beds, also relieves stiffness in joints.

- Grind poppy seeds *(khus-khus)* in sesame oil *(til ke tel)* and apply to the affected joints. Cover this with castor leaves and tie a bandage.

- Make a paste of 2 tablespoons dried ginger powder *(saunth)* with a little water. Heat it and apply it to rheumatic swellings of joints. The swelling and pain will subside.

- Massage the affected parts of your limbs with lemon juice mixed in coconut oil. Wet painful joint in warm water first; pat dry and then apply/rub the mix.

- In case of aching limbs with no one to press or massage them, take a rolling pin *(belan)* and roll it over your limbs.

Dos & Don'ts about the diet.

- Diet should be low in fat, protein and salt.
- Avoid milk & buttermilk.
- Avoid coffee, tea, alcohol, smoking & processed foods.
- Weight reduction is mandatory for overweight people.
- Take plenty of citrus fruits, fruit juices, fruits, vegetables & salads.

ASTHMA

What is Asthma?

Asthma is a condition where respiratory tracks become irritated and inflamed, and produce extra mucus. Breathing becomes difficult due to blockage.

Causes...

The exact cause of asthma is not very clear. However infections like flu and cold, pollution, chemical reactions, certain medicines, stress, could lead to asthma.

Symptoms...

Tightness in your chest, Coughing, Wheezing and Breathlessness.

Remedy (Nuskhe)...

❑ Drink water kept overnight in a copper vessel. This water, with traces of copper in it, is believed to change one's constitutional tendency to get respiratory problems.

❑ Take a pinch of cinnamon (dalchini) powder mix it with a little honey and take it every night. It acts like an expectorant in asthma.

❑ Boil 2-3 flakes garlic (lasan) in ¼ cup of milk and give it to the patient as a cure during the early stages of asthma.

❑ Chew on a piece of ginger (adrak) all throughout the day to relieve asthma, coughs, cold and sore throats.

❑ During the attack, mustard oil (sarson ka tel) mixed with a little camphor (kapoor) should be massaged over the back. This will loosen up phlegm and ease breathing.

❑ Boil carom seeds (ajwain) in water and inhale the steam.

❑ Add a handful of drumstick leaves (sahijan) to 1 cup water. Boil. Simmer on low flame for 3-4 minutes. Cool and strain. Add salt, pepper and lemon juice to taste. Drink once or twice everyday.

- Mix ¼ teaspoon asafoetida *(hing)*, 2 teaspoons honey, ½ teaspoon juice of betel leaf *(paan ka patta)* and ½ teaspoon white onion juice. Have it 2-3 times a day. To take out juice from betel leaf, crush to a paste and squeeze through a clean muslin cloth. For onion juice, grate the onion and squeeze through a clean muslin cloth.

- A very effective remedy for asthma is prepared by boiling 6 cloves *(laung)* in 3 tablespoons of water. Take 1 teaspoon of this decoction with a little honey, thrice daily. This is a very good expectorant.

- Mix equal amounts of fresh ginger *(adrak)* juice, honey & pomegranate *(anaar)* juice. Take 1 tablespoon, 1-2 times a day.

- Figs *(anjeer)* are known to drain the phlegm *(balgam)*. Take 3-4 dry figs, wash them well with warm water. Soak overnight in a cup of water. Eat them first thing in the morning and also drink the water. Do this for at least 2 months.

- Drinking a decoction of the seeds of amla, once or twice a day, proves very beneficial in the treatment of all respiratory disorders including Aasthma and Bronchitis.

Diet for an Asthmatics

- Avoid milk, milk products as they cause phlegm & lead to congestion in the lungs.

- Avoid citrus fruits (sour fruits), cold foods, ice-creams & deep fried food.

- Take plenty of fruits & vegetables with a high fibre content e.g. papaya, apples, watermelon.

- Avoid rice for dinner.

- Early dinner is best suited for these people. It ensures complete digestion before retirement.

- 1 teaspoon honey in a glass of hot water before bed time relaxes the throat by clearing accumulated phlegm in throat.

- Stay away from dusty places & avoid pets, particularly dogs.

Suggested Water Therapy for Asthmatics:

First thing in the morning, heat 3-4 glasses of water to which 2-3 teaspoon salt (white rock salt) has been added. Make it as warm as you can drink. *Sit on your haunches (hips) with heels on the floor.* Press your navel with your thumb/finger and drink this water. Drink as much as you can — so much that it causes vomiting. Vomit out. If not, poke your finger in your throat and vomit out. Do this *every* morning on an empty stomach for 1-2 months. Your asthma will surely get cured. Pregnant women or breast feeding mothers should not try this.

ASTHMA IN CHILDREN

Grind 5 tulsi leaves to a fine paste. Add 1 teaspoon honey to it and give to the child *every* morning and *evening* for 3-4 weeks.

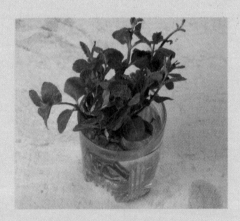

ALLERGIES

What is allergy?

When the body gets exposed to an antigen also known as allergen, a kind of abnormal tissue reaction takes place, which is referred to as allergy. Allergy can affect virtually any part of the body.

Causes...

An alergy is due to an environment or diet ingredient unsuited to a particular individual.

Symptoms...

Frequent headaches, High fever, Vomiting, Migraines, Dizziness, outbreak of Skin Rash, Eczema, Nervousness, Irritability, Swelling on the face and eyes, Asthma.

Remedy (Nuskhe)...

Banana is useful for a lot of people who suffer from allergies, like asthma, skin rash or stomach upsets. However some people may be allergic to bananas. Do not try this remedy if this be the case.

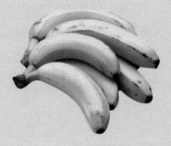

BACKACHE

What is backache?

When our back, for various reasons, is over-worked or strained and develops into a pain in the back region - it is called a backache. It can spread to the waist and hips also.

Causes...

Weak abdominal and back muscles, Incorrect posture, Muscular tension, Wrong diet, Lack of exercise, Kidney problems, Arthritis, Wearing of high heel shoes, Long hours of sitting.

Symptoms...

Pain felt in the middle of the back or in the lower back. When the pain gets aggravated, it tends to spread to both sides of the waist and hips.

Remedy (Nuskhe)...

- ❑ Massage back with turpentine oil *(tarpeen ka tel)*.
- ❑ Avoid rice, urad dal, maida and fried foods.
- ❑ Boil water with a few tulsi leaves or a black cardamom *(moti ilaichi)* for drinking.
- ❑ Eat 3-4 walnut halves *(akhrot giri)* every morning on an empty stomach for 1-2 weeks.

BAD BREATH OR HALITOSIS

What is halitosis?

Halitosis is a dental condition which causes bad breath.

Causes...

Certain foods, poor oral hygeine, mouth diseases, xerostomia (dry mouth), chewing tobacco products, hunger & stomach problems.

Symptoms...

Foul, odorous breath; an unpleasant taste in the mouth.

Remedy (Nuskhe)...

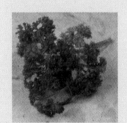

❑ Parsley leaves are rich in chlorophyll, nature's own deodoriser. Chew some leaves regularly and your breath will remain fresh. Alternatively, you can chew some cardamom seeds (*ilaichi*) to sweeten your breath.

❑ Chew some fennel seeds (*saunf*) frequently.

❑ Put a piece of cinnamon (*dalchini*) in a betel leaf (*paan ka patta*) and chew it.

❑ Boil some cinnamon (*dalchini*) in a cup of water. Store it in a clean bottle in your bathroom. Use it as a mouthwash frequently.

❑ Use neem twigs as tooth paste.

❑ Powder dried mint (*pudina*) leaves. Use as toothpowder.

BALDNESS

What is baldness?

When hair after falling does not growback, it is called baldness. Male baldness usually begins with thinning at the hairline, followed by the appearance of a bald spot on the crown of the head.

Women rarely develop bald patches. Instead, they experience a diffused thinning of their hair.

Causes...

Baldness is caused by a mix of genetics and hormones that we have a very little control on. The actual reason for baldness is still quite a mystery.

Symptoms...

Thinning or shedding of hair, breaking of hair, patchy bald areas (alopecia areata — an immune disorder causing temporary hair loss).

Remedy (Nuskhe)...

❑ Grind the remains of tobacco smoked in a hookah and add to boiling mustard oil. Cool and store. Massage on the bald patches regularly.

❑ Grind liquorice root pieces (*mulathi*). Add 1 tablespoon of this powder in 1 cup milk with ¼ teaspoon saffron (*kesar*). Apply this paste on bald patches at bedtime.

❑ Grind fenugreek seeds with water and apply on head. Leave for atleast 40 minutes before washing. Do it every morning for a month.

BED SORES

What are bed sores?

Bed sores are also called decubitus ulcers, pressure ulcers, or pressure sores.

Causes...

These tender or inflamed patches appear when skin remains pressed in one position and is unexposed to air for prolonged periods, for example, a bed ridden patient.

Remedy (Nuskhe)...

❑ Apply honey on the length and breadth of a banana leaf and lie on it for a few hours. Ensure its contact with the affected parts.

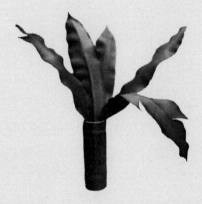

BED WETTING IN CHILDREN

What is bed wetting?

Bed-wetting or Enuresis is unconsciously urinating during the night. This condition is more common amongst children. Although most children between the ages of three and five begin to stay dry at night, the age at which children are physically and emotionally ready to have bladder control differs.

Causes...

Continual bed-wetting could be related to two things: A) a physically and/or neurologically weak bladder. B) a deep sleeping pattern. C) an inherited condition.

Symptoms...

No control over the bladder function specially at night. In adults, loss of bladder control is often referred to as urinary incontinence. This is found in patients with late-stage Alzheimer's disease or other forms of **dementia**. It is seen that bedwetting in children eventually subsides when children grow up. However some times children need behavioral or physiological treatment to be cured.

Remedy (Nuskhe)...

❑ Give 2 walnut halves (*akhrot giri*) and 5 raisins (*kishmish*) to the child before sleeping for 10-12 days.

BLACKHEADS

What are blackheads?

During adolescence most people likely deal with one form of acne or another, and one of the most common forms that plagues the most is blackheads.

Causes...

Black-heads are caused by over active oil producing glands (sebaceous glands) of the skin. The excess secretion of oil expands and thickens the pores of the skin. The oil collects in the pores and hardens into a plug. The pores are then clogged with hardened sebum or oil. Since the pores are open, the tip of the clogged grease is exposed to the air and oxidizes, turning black. Hence the name black-heads.

Symptoms...

Blackheads are dark spots that develop on the surface of the skin. Usually, they take place on the forehead, nose, and chin. But otherwise, they can appear on any part of the face. Severe blackheads lead to acne.

Remedy (Nuskhe)...

❑ Mix 1 teaspoon lemon juice in 1 teaspoon finely ground cinnamon (*dalchini*) powder and apply on affected areas frequently.

❑ Mix 1 teaspoon each turmeric (*haldi*) powder and juice of fresh coriander (*dhania*) leaves and apply daily as a face pack before going to sleep.

BLADDER STONES

What are bladder stones?

Bladder stones are crystalline masses that form from the minerals and proteins which naturally occur in urine. Bladder stones can form anywhere in the urinary tract before depositing in the bladder. They begin as tiny granules, about the size of a grain of sand, but they can grow to more than an inch in diameter. These stones can block the flow of urine causing pain and difficulty with urination. They can also scratch the bladder wall, which may lead to bleeding or infection.

Causes...

Age, Poor fluid intake, Incomplete emptying of the bladder, Recurrent urine infections, Medical conditions, for example, gout. Men are more prone to developing bladder stones.

Symptoms...

- Blood in the urine.
- Difficulty and pain while passing urine, extra pressure required to pass urine.
- Frequent urge to pass urine.

Remedy (Nuskhe)...

❑ Boil 2 figs (*anjeer*) in 1 cup of water. Drink daily for a month.

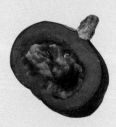

BLOOD DEFICIENCY

Remedy (Nuskhe)...

❑ Take 2 teaspoons of *amla* juice and mix it with two teaspoonfuls each of honey and lime. Add 1 teacup water and drink on an empty stomach every morning. Whenever fresh fruits are not available, dried *amla* can be used. Soak 1 tablespoon the previous night in a cup of water. (*Note*: The treatment should continue for at least 120 days to achieve expected results.)

❑ Soak 2 or 3 dried figs (*anjeer*) in 1 teacup water. Eat them along with milk next morning for a month.

BLOOD PRESSURE-HIGH

What is high blood pressure?

High blood pressure or hypertension means high pressure (tension) in the arteries. The arteries carry blood from the pumping heart to all the tissues and organs of the body. Blood pressure is considered normal when the machine reads below 120/80. When it reads 140/90 or more, it is considered to be high blood pressure.

Causes...

Too much salt intake, stress, genetic pool, hyperactive lifestyles are known to cause high BP. High BP leads to major health problems like heart attacks, kidney failure, strokes and vision impairment.

Symptoms...

The symptoms of high blood-pressure are weakness, restlessness, sleeplessness, head-ache, dizziness, vertigo, easy fatigue, frequent blushing accompained by rumbling of the bowels, palpitation of the heart, sweating, nausea and blurred vision. Sometimes there are no symptoms, that is why it is called a silent killer. Regular chekups are very important.

Remedy (Nuskhe)...

❑ Restrict salt intake & drink plenty of fluids (at least 8-10 glasses of water daily).

❑ Have a single pod garlic (*lasan*), one pod first thing every morning or if this is not available, have 1-2 cloves of ordinary garlic (*lasan*). If you get discomfort with having garlic first thing in the morning, swallow 2 cloves twice a day with water, any time or with meals.

❑ Mix 1 teaspoon honey, 1 teaspoon ginger (*adrak*) juice and 1 teaspoon cumin (*jeera*) powder. Have twice a day.

❑ Drink curry leaves (*curry patta*) juice 3 times a day (1 glassful) for 1-2 months and then reduce to only once in the morning. Have it on empty stomach. For taking out juice, fill your mixer with washed curry leaves, add ½ - ¾ glass water. Churn well and sieve. Add ½ - 1 lemon juice and drink fresh. This is one of the most effective remedies for lowering B.P.

❑ Drink coriander (*dhania*) juice made from fresh *dhania* 3 times a day.

❑ High blood-pressure can be cured by the daily intake of ¼ tsp pepper powder mixed with ¼ cup curd, first thing in the morning on an empty stomach for 48 days.

❑ Boil 1 cup leaves of drumsticks *(sahijan)* in about 2 glasses of water till the leaves are soft. Strain and cool. Drink the water on an empty stomach in the morning.

❑ Have a ripe papaya every day on an empty stomach and do not eat anything for 2 hours after that.

- People suffering from high B.P are advised to go on an apple diet for a few days.

- Have 1 cup of butter milk, to which 1 teaspoon of lemon juice has been added, as frequently as possible to bring down your B.P. Watermelon is high in potassium but very low in sodium and hence helps in lowering B.P. Eat as much as possible.

- Research has shown that high blood-pressure can be cured by eating the kernel out of the seeds of water-melon *(tarbooz giri)*. Have ½ tsp of it early morning.

- Having rice, particularly brown rice as the main staple food is very beneficial. As rice has very low sodium content and low cholesterol, it is a perfect diet for those who have been advised to have low salt diets.

- Consumption of natural diuretics like coconut water and butter milk helps lower B.P.

- Fruits such as mausami, orange, peaches *(aaru)*, plum *(aloo bukhara)*, are also beneficial.

- Last but not the least, rest, relaxation and good sleep are effective in keeping B.P. under control.

Banish BP: 6-3-6 Tension Formula

- Try the 6-3-6 formula for instant relaxation when you are tense or anxious. Slowly inhale to the count of 6 and hold your breath for a count of 3 and then exhale to the count of 6. This type of rhythmic breathing can control stress.

BLOOD PRESSURE – LOW

What is low blood pressure?

Low blood pressure is low flow of blood through the arteries and veins. This can cause damage to vital organs such as the brain, heart, and kidneys. If blood pressure drops to 100/60 it is low.

Causes...

Some of the causes are poor diet, dehydration, nausea, fever, heat stroke, anaemia or heriditary.

Symptoms...

Main symptoms are fainting, dizziness and fatigue.

Remedy (Nuskhe)...

❑ Healthy balanced diet of protein, carbohydrates, fats and sugar.

❑ Have the juice of 10-15 basil (*tulsi*) leaves mixed with 1 teaspoon honey. Crush the leaves to a paste and squeeze out the juice through a muslin cloth.

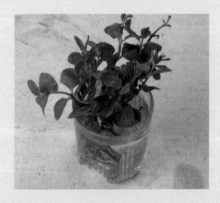

BODY WEAKNESS

Causes...

Poor diet, diabetes, anaemia.

Symptoms...

Lethargy, low evergy levels, fatigue, low resistance towards bacteria borne ailments.

Remedy (Nuskhe)...

❑ Soak 8 to 10 almonds and 1 teaspoon rice overnight. Remove the outer skin of almonds. Grind into a fine paste. Mix in some milk and a pinch of turmeric powder (*haldi*). Boil and drink along with sugar candy (*mishri*) or ordinary sugar to taste.

❑ Cut a mango into slices and place then on a platter. Sprinkle the following on mango slices: a pinch of saffron (*kesar*), cardamom (*chhoti illaichi*) and rose water (*gulab jal*) and 1 teaspoon honey. Take twice daily.

BOILS

What are boils?

A boil generally starts as a reddened, tender area. Over time, the area becomes firm and hard. Eventually, the center of the abscess softens and becomes filled with infection-fighting white blood cells that the body sends from the blood stream to eradicate the infection. This collection of white blood cells, bacteria, and proteins is known as pus. Finally, the pus forms a "head," which can be surgically opened or drained out through the surface of the skin.

Causes...

Ingrown hair, splinter or other foreign material that has become lodged in the skin, acne, clogged sweat glands that become infected.

Symptoms...

Infection or abscess on the skin.

Remedy (Nuskhe)...

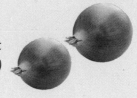

- ❏ Slightly roast a big onion on a naked flame. Mash it and mix in 1 teaspoon each turmeric powder *(haldi)* and ghee. Apply and tie a bandage.

- ❏ Mash some garlic flakes *(lasan)* and apply externally.

- ❏ Grind neem leaves to a paste and apply on affected parts.

- ❏ Apply a paste of 1 teaspoon ginger powder *(saunth)* and 1 teaspoon turmeric powder *(haldi)* on boils.

- ❏ Grind some black cumin *(kala jeera)* seeds in a little water and apply the paste on the affected areas.

- ❏ Heat black pepper powder in ½ teaspoon ghee until charred. Use this as an ointment.

- ❏ Take fenugreek leaf (*methi patta*) paste, heat it and when lukewarm, apply on the affected parts of the body.

- ❏ Soak bread in warm milk and sandwich the mixture in-between the folds of a clean cotton cloth. Apply this poultice to the boil and hold in place with a cotton bandage. This draws the dirt to the surface of the skin and simultaneously bursts the boil.

BRONCHITIS IN CHILDREN

What is bronchitis?

Bronchitis generally refers to an acute inflammation of the air passages within your lungs. It occurs when the wind pipe is blocked with mucus caused by infection etc. This causes acute coughing and breathing difficulties.

Causes...

Flu viruses, pneumonia, pollution, lung irritants, sudden change in temperature, prolonged cold and cough.

Symptoms...

Coughing, Shortness of breath, Frequent lung and respiratory tract infections, Wheezing.

Remedy (Nuskhe)...

❑ Mix 1 teaspoon garlic oil (*lasan*) and 3 teaspoons honey and give a small amount three times a day to the child.

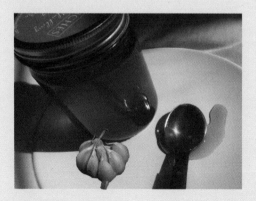

BURNS

What is a burn?

A burn is damage to your body's skin surface and tissues.

Causes...

Caused by heat, chemicals, electricity, sunlight or radiation.

Symptoms...

Pain, immediate redness of skin, which may develop into blisters and swelling.

Remedy (Nuskhe)...

❑ Cold water, and plenty of it, can sharply cut down the degree of burns. Contrary to popular belief it is not any greasy ointment or a blanket which provides relief to a burn victim, but soaking the burnt limb in cold water which is the best first aid. People have to be made aware of this simple yet effective method of dealing with burns, both superficial and deep.

❑ If it is burns from hot liquids then rub the affected area immediately with ice cubes and then apply a solution of milk and honey. This prevents formation of blisters.

❑ In the case of burns due to your clothes catching fire, apply generously a solution of freshly prepared very strong black tea which has been cooled to body temperature or pour cold water.

❑ Burn a handful of mango leaves to ashes and apply this on the affected parts.

❑ Mash a ripe banana well so as to form a smooth paste. Apply on wounds and burns and tie a cloth bandage on it for immediate relief.

❑ Desi ghee.

For Minor Burns: Remedy (Nuskhe)...

❑ For slight burns the application of honey or ink will reduce the burning sensation.

❑ Soda bicarb made into a very thin paste eases pain of burns (sunburns as well) if applied at once.

❑ The best way to treat a small burn at home is to apply toothpaste on the burnt area. The chemical in the toothpaste helps to soothe and does not allow blisters to form.

BURN SCARS

What are burn scars?

These scars that appear after a burn injury has healed completely.

Causes...

Burns.

Symptoms...

White or pink wrinkled skin surface, visibly different from normal body complexion.

Remedy (Nuskhe)...

Boil 1 cup neem bark (*neem ki khal*) in 4 cups water. Remove from fire and shake liquid. Apply the emerging froth on the affected area. Repeat several times and for several days.

BRUISES

What is a bruise?

Skin discolouration to blue or black accompanied by pain.

Causes...

Normally a sudden, hard impact on a body part by a hard or abrasive surface causes a bruise.

Symptoms...

Skin surface turns blue or blue back and is painful to touch or move.

Remedy (Nuskhe)...

Slice a raw onion & place over the bruise. Do not apply this to broken skin.

BLEEDING GUMS

❑ If you have bleeding wounds in between the teeth, insert a little cotton moistened with sandalwood oil *(chandan ka tel)* at the affected spots or you can add a few drops of sandalwood oil to your milk or coffee or tea, and drink it daily for 10-15 days.

❑ Mix a little powdered alum *(phitkari)* with a little honey to form a thick paste and rub the teeth and gums with this mixture.

CATARACT, EARLY STAGES

What is Cataract?

Cataract is an eye disease, it happens when the lens of the eye becomes opaque.

Causes...

- Diabetes, Metabolic disorders, Ageing
- Heredity
- Use of steroids
- Trauma, Exposure to radiation
- Alcohol, Smoking

Symptoms...

Problem with bright light, blurred vision, double vision, pupil discoloured to whitish grey, colours dimming, affected night vision, difficulty in reading.

Remedy (Nuskhe)...

- ❑ Mix 1 teaspoon rose water (*gulab jal*) with 1 teaspoon fresh lemon juice. Add 10 drops of this to the eyes.

- ❑ Soak 10-12 almonds in a cup of water overnight. Next morning remove skin and grind the almonds with 10-12 peppercorns (*sabut kaali mirch*) to a paste. Add a cup of water and honey or sugar to taste. Drink once daily. Continue for a few weeks.

CHEST CONGESTION CAUSING BREATHING PROBLEMS

What is chest congestion?

Blockage in the chest which reduces free flow of oxygen to the lungs.

Causes...

Sudden change in temperature, phlegm.

Symptoms...

Laboured breathing, sometimes cold and cough also, body ache.

Remedy (Nuskhe)...

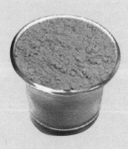

- ❑ Grind ¼ teaspoon mustard seeds (*sarson*) to a smooth paste. Mix with honey and eat.

- ❑ Mix equal quantities of mustard powder (*sarson*) and rice flour. Add some water and boil until it reaches a paste-like consistency. Spread on a handkerchief and foment the chest and neck when bearably hot.

- ❑ Add to ½ litre (2½ cups) of boiling water, 1 teaspoon carom seeds (*ajwain*) powder and 1 teaspoon turmeric (*haldi*) powder. Cool. Take 1 tablespoon of this mixture along with 1 teaspoon honey.

CHOLESTEROL, HIGH

What is cholesterol?

Identified as a waxy, fat like substance that lines all cell walls of our body, cholesterol produces many hormones, vitamin D, and bile acids that help to digest fat in the body. Too much cholesterol in the body leads to deposits on the inside of the arteries of the heart, mostly leading to heart diseases.

Causes...

Overweight, hereditary, diet, age.

Symptoms...

High cholesterol doesn't have any symptoms. The only way to know if you have high cholesterol is to get it checked through a simple blood test, called a fasting lipoprotein profile.

Remedy (Nuskhe)...

☐ Sunflower seeds contain a substantial amount of linoleic acid, which is helpful in reducing cholesterol deposits on the walls of the arteries. Using sunflower seed oil in the condition of high cholesterol is thus recommended.

☐ Finely dice an onion and mix it with 1 cup buttermilk along with ¼ teaspoon black pepper (*kali mirch*) powder and drink.

☐ Regularly intake coriander (*dhania*) decoction made by boiling 2 teaspoons dry coriander seed (*dhania*) powder in 1 cup water. (Milk and sugar can be added to improve its taste. This could be a welcome substitute for tea or coffee.)

☐ Onion juice is very helpful in reducing cholesterol. Mix 1 tsp onion juice with 1 tsp honey. Have it once a day.

- Eating cooked bottle gourd *(lauki)* is good for people having this condition.
- Increase the intake of raw garlic as it helps to reduce cholesterol.
- Eating the kernel of the seeds of water-melon *(tarbooz giri)* reduces cholesterol. Have ½ tsp of *tarbooz giri* early morning, every day.

COLD

What is cold?

A viral infectious disease of the upper respiratory system (nose and throat).

Causes...

Viral infection, sudden change in temperature, long exposure to a cold environment.

Symptoms...

Running nose, frequent sneezing, feverishness, body ache, head ache.
Nasal congestion, scratchy, sore or phlegmy throat.

Remedy (Nuskhe)...

- The juice of two lemons in ½ a litre (2½ cups) of boiling water sweetened with honey, taken at bed time, is a very effective remedy.
- Have ginger *(adrak)* tea. Cut ginger into 1" – 1½" pieces and boil with a cup of water. Give 8-10 boils. Strain, sweeten with ½ teaspoon sugar and drink hot.
- A tablespoon of carom seeds *(ajwain)* crushed and tied up in a muslin cloth can be used for inhalation to relieve congestion/blocked nose.
- A teaspoon of cumin seeds *(jeera)* is added to 1 glass of boiling water. Strain and simmer for a few minutes. Let it cool. Drink it 1-2 times a day.

If sore throat is also present, add a few small pieces of dry ginger (*adrak*) to the boiling water.

❏ Six pepper corns (*sabut kali mirch*) finely ground and mixed with a glass of warm water, sweetened with 5-6 *batashas* (a variation of sugar candy) can be taken for a few nights.

❏ In the case of acute cold, boil 1 tablespoon pepper powder in a cup of milk along with a pinch of turmeric (*haldi*) and have once daily for at least 3 days.

❏ People prone to cold should consume guava throughout winters. This will protect them from cold throughout the year. This is because of the high content of vitamin C present in the guava.

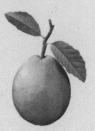

COUGH

What is cough?

Constriction in the throat which obstructs normal breathing.

Causes...

Consumption of cold or sour food by people with sensitive throats, phlegm, certain allergies, sudden chage in temperature.

Symptoms...

Frequent need to clear irritation in throat or phelgm in the chest by forceful and noisy exittance of air through the mouth.

Remedy (Nuskhe)...

- To stay away from cough of all kinds, boil some fresh basil (*tulsi*) leaves in 2 cups water. Continue to boil till reduced to 1 cup. Drink this water every morning.

- The high pectin content of apples relieves cough and helps in eliminating toxins from the body. A minimum of 300-350 gms of apples or their juice should be consumed daily for 8-10 days for beneficial results.

- Mix 1 teaspoon of honey with ½ tsp ground liquorice (*mulethi*) and take it twice a day for any type of cough.

- For night coughs, mix 1 teaspoon honey in a cup of hot drink (milk or tea) before bed time.

- Drink turmeric (*haldi*) powder boiled in milk at bed time. Boil 1 cup milk. After the boil, reduce heat and add ½ teaspoon *haldi* powder. Keep on low heat for 2 minutes. Remove from fire.

- If there is a lot of mucus (*balgam*) with cough, take 10 peppercorns (*sabut kali mirch*), 4 small sticks of liquorice (*mulethi*) and 2 teaspoons of sugar candy (*mishri*); pound together to a fine powder and have ¼ teaspoon four times a day.

- Consume a mix of ½ teaspoon carom seeds (*ajwain*) with ½ teaspoon honey and 1 crushed peppercorn (*sabut kali mirch*).

- Powder 1 clove (*laung*). Add a pinch of sugar and 1 teaspoon honey. Let the child lick it little by little.

- Mix equal amounts of honey and ginger (*adrak*) juice. For better results warm the mixture a little & then have it. Have 1 teaspoon, 2-3-4 times a day.

- Three pepper corns (*saboot kali mirch*) with a pinch of black cumin (*shah jeera*) and a pinch of salt gives relief.

- Mix 1 teaspoon pepper powder with 4 teaspoon jaggery (*gur*). Make small balls. Suck 3-4 balls/tablets during the day.

- Give 1 teaspoon of basil (*tulsi*) leaves juice, 2-3 times a day to children having cough. Tulsi leaves can be crushed to a paste and the paste squeezed through a clean muslin cloth to get juice.

- Heat ½ cup of mustard oil (*sarson ka tel*). Add 5 flakes of garlic *(lasan)* and let it turn black. Take it off the fire and let it cool. Bottle it and use it to massage nose, head and chest.

- Keep 5 whole peppercorns (*sabut kali mirch*) in your mouth before sleeping. Do not crush. You will sleep undistrubed. Crush and swallow in the morning.
- Grind tulsi leaves and 1" piece ginger. Extract juice. Mix with 6 tbsp honey. Take 1 tsp of this three times a day for a few days.

COUGH (DRY)

- Mix 8-10 tablespoons of coconut milk with 1 tablespoon poppy seeds (*khus khus*) and 1 tablespoon pure honey. Take every night before going to bed.

COUGH WITH PHLEGM *(BALGAM)*

- Mix equal amounts of onion juice & honey. Have 1 teaspoon, 3-4 times a day. This is a preventive medicine against cold in winter.
- Lemon juice has the property of dislodging phlegm. It's consumption pulls out the phlegm and cures cough.
- Take 8-10 *tulsi* leaves and wash well. To 1 cup of water, add these tulsi leaves, 1-2 cloves of garlic (*lasan*), ½" piece ginger, crushed, and 4-5 peppercorns (*sabut kali mirch*). Boil the water and keep simmering on fire till the quantity is reduced to ¼ cup. Cool. Strain. Add 1 teaspoon honey. Drink this every morning.
- Crush ¼ cup of carom seeds (*ajwain*) and tie in a thin muslin cloth (*malmal*) and place it near the child's pillow.

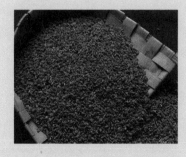

CONGESTION (PHLEGM OR BALGAM) ONLY

Remedy (Nuskhe)...

❑ For phlegm congestion, take out 1 cup juice of fenugreek leaves *(methi leaves)*. To take out juice, wash leaves well and blend in a mixer with a little water. Strain. Add 1 tsp ginger *(adrak)* juice and 1 tsp honey to this and drink it 2-3 times a day.

❑ Gargle with hot salted water, or hot black salted tea water.

COLIC IN BABIES

What is colic?

Trapped gas in the body.

Causes...

Lactose intolerance, allergies, immature digestive system exposure to cold, constipation.

Symptoms...

Severe pain in the stomach. Hard and tight stomach, constipation, irritability and restlessness.

Remedy (Nuskhe)...

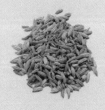

❑ Boil a teaspoon of fennel seeds *(saunf)* in a cup of water. Boil for 2-3 minutes and keep it to cool for 15-20 minutes. Strain. Add 1-2 teaspoon to every feed of milk of the baby. It helps cure colic.

CONSTIPATION

'A healthy stomach is a healthy body.' Many diseases have their roots in the digestive system.

Never take laxatives too often or for too long for the cure of constipation. They will weaken the intestines and the faculty of natural bowel movement. They will ultimately lead to damage of the inner walls of intestines resulting in dysentery, intestinal wounds and ultimate development of piles. Instead eat a fibre rich diet of raw fruits and vegetables as salads, have plenty of water, and some exercise.

What is constipation?

Constipation is a common gastrointestinal complaint. People who are constipated may find it difficult and painful to have regular bowel movement.

Causes...

- Insufficient fibre in diet. Less fluid intake. Lack of exercise. Certain Medications.
- Changes in life or routine such as pregnancy, old age, and travel.
- Ignoring the bowel movement.

Symptoms...

Bloated feeling in the stomach, discomfort, general unease due to gas.

Remedy (Nuskhe)...

- Drink a hot glass of water with 1 teaspoon honey and juice of ½ a lemon first thing in the morning.

- Drink one litre (4 glasses) of water first thing in the morning.

- Soak 6-8 dates (*khajoor*) in a cup of water at night. Churn in the mixer in the morning & drink first thing in the morning.

- A cup of hot milk at night before going to bed.

- Chew a few liquorice (*mulethi*) sticks. One of its many properties is that it is a natural laxative.

- Soak 6-8 raisins (*kishmish*) in hot water. When cool, crush well and strain. When given routinely even to little infants, it helps to regulate bowel movement (however care should be taken so as not to give too much or the child might get loose motions.)

- Consume 6-8 apricots (*khurmani*) a day.

- Bulk forming vegetables like carrots, radish, spinach, cabbage or roughage creating diet should be consumed. Instead of juice always opt for eating the fruit.

- Whole wheat flour should be used and processed foods (*maida*, cheese, confectionery) should be avoided.

- Taking 2-3 teaspoons of *isabgol* in milk or warm water either first thing in the morning or at bed time is very beneficial.

- Have your meals at fixed time. Drink a glass of hot water half an hour before breakfast and half an hour before retiring at night. Make a habit of answering calls of nature at fixed time every day.

- Take 1 cup of bottle gourd (*lauki*) juice . Add a little salt to it and drink it daily for some days. This will cure chronic constipation.

- Almonds being laxative in nature are very beneficial for constipation. Soak 3-4 almonds with 2-3 dried figs (*anjeer*) in a cup of water in the morning. At night remove the skin of almonds and grind both almonds and figs to a paste. Add a little honey and have this at bedtime for a few days, to facilitate clear motions next morning.

- As the figs contain a large cellulose content and a thick skin, they are very beneficial in the treatment of constipation. Soak 2-3 dried figs in 1 cup water. Next morning add 1 tablespoon of honey and consume these along with the water in which they were soaked. Continue for at least 1 month. Consumption of fresh figs is also beneficial in curing constipation.

- Consumption of grapefruit helps in relieving constipation as it supplies bulk to facilitate bowel movement.

- Daily consumption of grapes is highly recommended for people suffering from constipation. The organic acids (malic, citric and tartaric acids) present in grapes in combination with the sugar and cellulose, stimulate the activity of the bowels, thus curing constipation. A minimum of 300-400 gms of grapes or their juice should be taken daily.

- Guava is a mild laxative. It is good to have it for breakfast.

- Amla is a laxative fruit hence its regular use will help to overcome the problem of habitual constipation. Soak 2-3 dried amlas in water overnight. Next morning, mash them and sieve them. Add a little honey (1-2 teaspoons) and drink this first thing in the morning.

- Consuming 3-4 oranges a day or drinking orange juice daily will take care of this problem. The best way to have oranges for this problem is at breakfast and before retiring at night.

- Daily consumption of papaya is a sure way of getting rid of constipation. In addition, its regular consumption also cures bleeding piles, chronic dysentery and hyperacidity.

- The fibrous element of sweet lime proves beneficial in overcoming the problem of constipation. It is recommended to eat the fruit and not have its juice when suffering from constipation.

- Watermelon is mildly laxative in nature. Regular consumption of the fruit takes care of any constipation that you might be suffering. 2 medium sized bowls of the fruit should be had daily.

CRAMPS

What are cramps?

Unpleasant, often painful sensations, usually of muscles.

Causes..

- Cold or overexertion
- Illness
- Lack of salt and water (electrolyte disturbance)
- Hypothyroidism

Remedy (Nuskhe)...

- ❑ Apply clove oil (*laung ka tel*) on the affected parts.
- ❑ Eating foods high in potassium, such as bananas, prunes and potatoes.
- ❑ Soft massage on the cramped muscle, stretching the muscle and dipping the part in hot water to which some salt has been added. Heat improves superficial blood circulation and makes muscle more flexible.

CUTS, SCRATCHES AND WOUNDS

What are cuts?

A type of wound, usually a laceration or incision into the skin.

Causes...

Contact with sharp or pointed objects like knives or thorns, any injury, accident, falling or slipping.

Symptoms...

Swelling or bleeding, severe pain in that area.

Remedy (Nuskhe)...

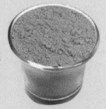

❑ Continuous flow of blood from cuts and wounds can be stopped quickly by pressing the place with a little turmeric *(haldi)* powder which is also an antiseptic.

❑ If you get wounds or cuts and start bleeding profusely, apply coffee powder at once on the injured area.

❑ A cotton plug dipped in brandy and dabbed on the wound acts as an antiseptic.

❑ In the event of wounds due to falls, cuts etc., crush a betel leaf *(pan ka patta)* with lime *(nimbu)* juice and apply it on the affected parts.

❑ Application of the milk got by breaking the leaves or twigs of pipal tree to abrasions, cuts etc. will cure them very quickly. This is also effective in the successful treatment of fissures on the sides of heels and feet.

❑ All kinds of wounds and cuts can be speedily cured by the application of honey. Even the scar of the wound will disappear.

CANCER

What is cancer?

A disease characterized by a population of cells that grow and divide without respect to normal limits, invade and destroy adjacent tissues and may spread to other parts. The growth of cells can either result to benign or malignant (cancerous) tumour. The benign may tend to become malignant over passage of time.

Causes...

Carcinogens such as tobacco-smoking, radiation, chemicals.

Symptoms...

- 7 warning signals in recognising the presence of cancer
- Change in bowel or bladder habits
- A sore that does not heal
- Unusual bleeding or discharge
- Thickening or lump in the breast or elsewhere
- Indigestion or difficulty in swallowing
- Obvious changes in a wart or mole
- A nagging cough or hoarseness.

Remedy (Nuskhe)...

- ❑ Almonds have a rich composition and favourable influence on the calcium balance and the defence mechanism of our bodies. They are therefore highly recommended for consumption in the diet of a cancer patient.
- ❑ Banana possesses an excellent potassium-sodium balance (proportion) and that is very important in the diet of a cancer patient.

- Of all the foodstuffs, coconut contains the largest amount of *selenium*, which is an important part of an enzyme present in the human body. This enzyme is very important in the metabolic process of poly unsaturated fatty acids and prevents the development of free radicals. Hence, coconut consumption is very beneficial in cases of cancer.

- Papaya contains different types of enzymes due to which it is said to be effective in the treatment of cancer.

- Pineapples have an alkaline reaction in our bodies. It is the most essential foodstuff in the cancer diet. In fact it is included in the menu everyday. It is said that if you go on an exclusive pineapple diet for one week every few months you will never get cancer. It is said to be a preventive against cancer.

  A. T. Hovannession of Iran in his book "Raw Eating" says that any kind of cancer can be cured by raw-eating; which means that the patient should eat only raw things whether they be fruits or vegetables or liquid. He says that raw eating in fact prevents and cures any disease and that a human being can live up to 140-150 years.

NATURE CURE THERAPY FOR CANCER

- Research has shown that grapes contain *ellagin acid*, one of the very highly recommended photo chemicals with a restraining influence on cancer. In the grape cure treatment for cancer, the patient is required to get his body cleansed thoroughly through nature cure treatment. He is asked to fast for 2-3 days on water alone and is also given an enema. On the day the grape cure starts, the patient is given 1-2 glasses of cold water in the morning. After an hour or so, a glass of grape juice is given. Then every 2 hours grape juice is given, 6-7 times in a day. So during the whole day 5-6 litres of grape juice is consumed by the patient. This treatment is known to cure cancer. This is continued for 1-2 weeks and if found helpful is continued longer. This treatment however should be undertaken only under the guidance and advice of an experienced naturopath.

CHOLERA

What is cholera?

A severe diarrheal disease caused by a virus.

Causes...

Transmission to humans is by ingesting contaminated water or food.

Symptoms...

Upset stomach, Massive watery diarrhoea, may include terrible muscle and stomach cramps, vomitting and fever in early stages.

Remedy (Nuskhe)...

- Coconut water is an indisputable remedy in cholera. In cases of cholera the patient on account of loose motions and vomiting loses a lot of body fluids and this can lead to dehydration. Coconut water, being rich in potassium and mineral, when given to cholera patients helps prevent 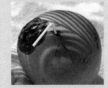 dehydration and also corrects the electrolyte balance of the body. In addition, as the water is antibacterial, it helps in expelling the cholera germs from the intestines.
- Boil 1 tsp cloves (*laung*) in 10 cups water till it is reduced to 5 cups. Take in draughts frequently.

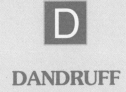

DANDRUFF

What is dandruff?

Dandruff's scientific name is *Pityriasis capitis.* It is the excessive flaking of dead skin that forms on the scalp.

Causes...

- Improper diets
- Constipation
- Harsh shampoos
- Exposure to cold

Symptoms...

- White flakes fall from head and find their place on eyebrows, shoulders and clothing.
- Itching

Remedy (Nuskhe)...

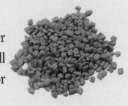

- ❑ Soak 2 tablespoon fenugreek seeds (*methi dana*) in water overnight. In the morning grind into a fine paste. Apply all over scalp and leave for ½ an hour. Wash with *Shikakai* or mild shampoo.
- ❑ Boil a handful of neem leaves in 4 teacups of water. After cooling and filtering use for rinsing hair.

DEAFNESS

What is deafness?

Refers to a physical condition characterized by lack of sensitivity to sound.

Causes...

* Genetic disorder - could be due to harmful drugs taken by mother during pregnancy.
* Infections from diseases like Meningitis, Mumps, Measles or ear infection.
* Injury or Accident.

Symptoms...

Impaired partial or total hearing.

Remedy (Nuskhe)...

❑ Use raw onion juice as ear drops.
❑ Put two drops of lukewarm neem oil inside the ear.

DEHYDRATION

What is dehydration?

Loss of water or insufficient water level in the body.

Causes...

Excessive vomitting, diarrhoea.

Symptoms...

Acute weakness which can be fatal if unattended.

Remedy (Nuskhe)...

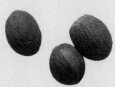

❑ Soak half a nutmeg (*jaiphal*) in 2 cups water for over 2-3 hours. Take 1 teaspoon of this infusion and mix in 1 cup fresh coconut water. Drink twice or thrice a day.

❑ Add ¼ teaspoon salt, 3 teaspoon brown sugar or ordinary sugar and 2 teaspoon lemon juice to 1 cup of water, mix well and drink.

DELIVERY OF BABIES MADE EASIER

❑ Pregnant women should freely take lemon juice sherbet (*nimboo paani*) from the 4th month onwards to ensure easy delivery.

❑ Some pregnant women get false pains during the 8th month itself. On such occasions grind a few coriander seeds (*sabut dhaniya*) with the water in which rice has been washed. Give 1 spoonful of this to the patient several times. The pains will subside and the womb will return to normal.

❑ Mix 3 teaspoon lemon juice, ¼ teaspoon powdered black pepper and 1 teaspoon honey in 1 cup water. Drink for 3 months.

❑ 1 tsp of desi ghee added to a glass of hot milk, consumed in the last month of pregnancy, makes delivery fast and easier.

❑ *To lighten the post delivery stretch marks on the body, apply olive oil after bath, on areas which are affected. You should start this treatment in the third month of pregnancy.*

DENTAL PROBLEMS

What are dental problems?

Problems relating to teeth or gums.

Causes...

Poor oral hygenic, chewing tobacco.

Symptoms...

Decaying teeth, swollen or bleeding gums, pain, excessive sensitivity to hot or cold food or liquids.

Remedy (Nuskhe)...

❑ Put ½ teaspoon of powdered rock salt (*sendha namak*) on the palm of your hand and add 1 teaspoon of mustard oil (*sarson ka tel*) to it. Mix well. Every night before going to bed massage the gums gently with this oil. Then rub the left over paste on the teeth lightly and immediately wash the mouth. If possible gargle a few times with warm water.

❑ Turmeric (*haldi*), burnt and finely powdered, can be used as toothpowder.

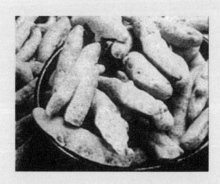

DEPRESSION

What is depression?

Inability to cope with changed circumstances.

Causes...

Sudden loss, unwanted change of environment.

Symptoms...

Loss of appetite, general disinterest, headache, bodyache.

Remedy (Nuskhe)...

❑ Boil ¼ teaspoon powdered cardamom (*chhoti ilaichi*) seeds in thin tea water and drink.

❑ Mix 1/8 teaspoon nutmeg (*jaiphal*) powder with 1 tablespoon freshly extracted amla juice. Take 3 times a day.

❑ Banana contains *serotonin*, a neurotransmitter that makes nerve contact possible. Lack of serotonin in the brain can result in depression and suicidal tendencies. Thus banana is a very important fruit in your daily diet.

❑ Watermelon consumption on a regular basis benefits people who are suffering from depression or who are prone to depression.

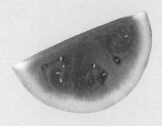

DIABETES

What is diabetes?

A disease in which the body does not produce or properly use insulin - a hormone that is needed to convert sugar, starches and other food into energy needed for daily life. Normal sugar level in blood should be 70 - 110 mg/dl. Increase of sugar count above 110 mg/dl is called diabetes.

Causes...

- Genetic factors - If one of your parents is a diabetic, your chances of being one by the time you turn 40, are 40%.

- Excessive consumption of alcohol, fats or sugar, overweight, drugs.

Symptoms...

The commonest symptoms of diabetes are unusual thirst, frequent urination, loss of weight despite increased appetite and food intake, weakness and drowsiness, reducing vision and often itching and boils. There is no absolute cure for diabetes; but it can be almost completely controlled.

Dadi maa recommends...

- ❑ For diabetes, diet restriction & light exercise like walking is a must as this controls the sugar level.

- ❑ A tablespoon of *amla* juice mixed with a cup of fresh bitter gourd (*karela*) juice taken daily for 2 months will reduce blood sugar.

- ❑ Dry tender leaves of the mango tree in shade. Powder and preserve them. Half a teaspoon of this powder twice a day in the morning and evening proves beneficial.

- ❑ Coarsely powder fenugreek seeds (*methi dana*) and have 1-2 teaspoons in the morning everyday. (Vary dosage according to individual tolerance level).

- Eating 10 fresh fully grown curry leaves (*kari patta*) every morning for 3 months is said to prevent diabetes due to heredity factors.

- Chew 8-10 basil (*tulsi*) leaves in the morning.

Guidelines of a Diabetics Diet:

- Use the following fruits and vegetables sparingly and with caution: carrots (*gajar*), peas (*matar*), beans, sweet potato (*shakarkandi*), beetroot (*chukandar*), potatoes, jackfruit (*kathal*), banana, grapes (*angoor*), cheeku, leechi, custard apple (*sharifa*), dry fruits, mango, raisins (*kishmish*).

- Eat plenty of vegetables like lettuce (*salaad patta*), tomato and fruits.

- Foods rich in fibre should be preferred.

- Daily intake of calories should be restricted.

- Use proteins moderately.

- Milk & nuts intake to be restricted to the minimum whereas have plenty of curd and buttermilk (*chhachh*).

- Avoid all refined foods & sweets.

- Drink 8-10 glasses of water daily.

- 3 grapefruits taken 3 times a day by a diabetic (one who is not on insulin) will help him to get his sugar under control. In the juice form it is recommended that a diabetic consumes ½ a litre of grape juice a day.

More Suggestions To Control Diabetes

❑ Grind 4 tender green leaves of jamun with ¼ cup water. Strain and drink early morning for 10 days. After this have it for 10 days after every 2 months. It controls urine sugar.

❑ Take 60 gm (½ cup) of good, ripe jamun. Boil 1½ cups water. Add the jamuns to it and keep covered for 30 minutes. Mash the fruit well after 30 minutes and strain. Divide it into 3 parts and have 1 part each time, thrice a day.

❑ Take the seeds of jamun and peel to get the kernel from the seeds (*guthli ki giri*). Dry these kernels in the shade and grind to a powder. Take every morning and evening, ½ teaspoon with fresh water. Continue taking for 21 days.

❑ Dry some neem leaves in the shade for 2 or 3 days, powder them and store in a jar. Before going to bed at night, dissolve 1 teaspoonful of this powder in hot milk together with a few pinches of powdered cumin (*jeera*) and carom seeds (*ajwain*) for 30 days or more.

❑ It is good for diabetic patients if they frequently eat bitter gourd *(karela)*. This will decidely control diabetes and its complications. Frequently drinking the juice out of the leaves of the bitter gourd vine is also as effective.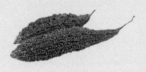

❑ Eating dates *(khajoor)* helps to control diabetes. The sweetness of dates is harmless to diabetic patients.

3 ways to prevent diabetes

❑ Normalise body weight in relation to age and height.

❑ Walk briskly at least 4 kms a day.

❑ Control alcohol intake, kick the smoking habit and reduce dependence on drugs.

DIARRHOEA

What is diarrhoea?

A condition in which the sufferer has frequent watery loose bowel movements.

Causes...

This condition can occur as a symptom of infection, allergy or food intolerance.

Symptoms...

Abdominal pain, nausea and vomitting

Remedy (Nuskhe)...

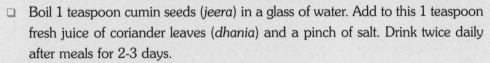

- Combine 1 teaspoon each powdered ginger (*adrak*), powdered cumin (*jeera*) and powdered cinnamon (*dalchini*) with honey and make into a thick paste. Take 1 teaspoon thrice daily.

- Boil 1 teaspoon cumin seeds (*jeera*) in a glass of water. Add to this 1 teaspoon fresh juice of coriander leaves (*dhania*) and a pinch of salt. Drink twice daily after meals for 2-3 days.

- Mash 1 ripe banana along with a pinch of salt and 1 teaspoon tamarind pulp (*imli ka gooda*). Take twice a day.

- Drinking a strong cup of unsweetened black tea is very effective for stopping diarrhoea.

- Peel an apple and shred it. Keep the shredded pieces in a plate for approximately 20 minutes until they turn brown in colour, and then eat them.

- Slice the tender unripe bel fruit. Sun dry them. Powder the slices. Take 1 teaspoon along with warm water twice a day.

- Take every night, 3 cloves of garlic (*lasan*), chopped and boiled in milk.

- Make a paste of 1 green chilli along with 2 tablespoon lemon juice & ½ teaspoon camphor (*kapoor*). Take ¼ teaspoon of this paste.

- 2 or 3 teaspoons coriander seeds (*sabut dhania*) soaked overnight in water and taken next morning with 1 cup buttermilk (*chhachh*) is beneficial.

- Boil ¼ teaspoon powdered cardamom (*chhoti ilaichi*) seeds in thin tea water and drink.

- Mix juice of 15-20 tender curry leaves (*curry patta*) with 1 teaspoon honey and drink.

- Apply ginger (*adrak*) juice around the navel.

- Soak a little rice in water for ½ hour. Strain rice. Roast rice in 1 tsp desi ghee. Add ½ tsp ajwain seeds. Cover with water. Cook to make kichdi. Eat this and nothing else at mealtimes.

DIARRHOEA DUE TO INDIGESTION OF FOOD

Remedy (Nuskhe)...

- Insert ¼ teaspoon nutmeg (*jaiphal*) powder inside a ripe banana and eat.

- Swallow 1 tsp fenugreek seeds *(methi daana),* without chewing along with 1 tbsp curd *(dahi)* for immediate relief from diarrhoea. In case the problem is acute, take it twice a day. While travelling, fenugreek seeds can be taken with water also.

- Boil 1 cup of water and add in 5-8 tender leaves of guava *(amrood)*. Boil for a further 2-3 minutes. Remove from fire and cover the pan and keep aside for another 5-10 minutes. Add a pinch of salt to the liquid before consuming. Drink as much as you can.

- Mix a little salt with juice of lemon (*nimbu*), drink it without diluting with water.

- Drink rice water "*kanji*" (the starch water which is left after boiling rice) mixed with some rock-salt (*kala namak*) and some roasted cumin seeds (*bhuna jeera*).

- Mix a pinch of salt with 1 tablespoon ginger juice and drink it every hour.

- Eat plums; plums control diarrhea and do not lead to constipation.

DYSENTERY

What is dysentery?

Infection of the digestive tract.

Causes...

Bacterial infection

Symptoms...

- Onset is usually abrupt with high fever, followed by vomitting, abdominal pain and diarrhoea.

- Stools sometimes tinged with blood.

Remedy (Nuskhe)...

- As soon as the disease starts, one should immediately avoid all the food stuffs which are responsible for the disease. Stale food, tamarind (*imli*), raw mangoes (aam), chillies, green vegetables, potatoes, gramflour, mawa, tea, coffee and fried eatables should be avoided.

- 1 teaspoon of powdered aniseeds (*saunf*) mixed with ½ teaspoon sugar should be taken thrice a day.

- Grind some curry leaves to a fine paste and mix this paste in ½ glass butter milk (*lassi*) and drink it 3 or 4 times a day. This cures dysentery and diarrhoea.

- The juice of pomegranate (*anar*) fruit is a well known remedy for mild diarrhoea and dysentery accompanied by a suitable diet.

- For dysentery, drink strong tea without milk or sugar.

- Dry ginger powder (*saunth*) mixed with buttermilk (*lassi*), if taken after meals will help.

- Eat Pomegranate. It is said to be useful in the control of dysentery (even diarrhoea).

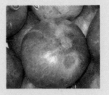

- The combination of ripe banana, salt and tamarind pulp is very effective in dysentery.

DIGESTIVE AND LIVER PROBLEMS

Remedy (Nuskhe)...

- Suck or eat a mango and then drink a glass of milk after it for a few days, to get maximum benefit in liver and digestive disorders.

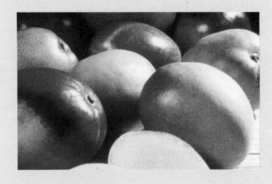

EAR

EAR ACHE

Remedy (Nuskhe)...

- ❑ Boil well 1 teaspoon lasan *(garlic)* in 2 tablespoons gingelly oil *(til ka tel)*. Cool and filter. Use as ear drops (2 to 3 drops).

- ❑ Mix a few drops of lemon juice in 1 teaspoon lukewarm water. Put 4 drops of this into the ear.

- ❑ Use neem leaf juice as ear drops.

- ❑ Peel 2 flakes of garlic *(lasan)* and mix with 2 tablespoon of mustard oil *(sarson ka tel)*. Heat on low flame. When the garlic starts burning and turns blackish, remove oil from fire. Strain through a clean muslin cloth. Dip a piece of cotton wool in warm oil and squeeze in 2-3 drops of oil into the ear.

- ❑ Put 3-4 drops of the juice extracted out of tulsi leaves.

- ❑ Warm ¼ teaspoon mustard oil *(sarson ka tel)* and pour it in th ear. Thereafter, dip a piece of cotton wool in the oil and plug it in the ear.

EARACHE ON FLIGHT (WHILE FLYING)

Remedy (Nuskhe)...

- ❑ To ease earache while traveling by air, close your mouth, hold your nose tight and blow your nose very gently. This trick equalizes the air pressure in the middle ear. Another way is to act as if you are swallowing something.

EAR BOILS (INNER EAR)

Remedy (Nuskhe)...

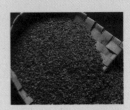

❑ Heat 2 teaspoons mustard oil. Add ½ teaspoon carom (*ajwain*) seeds and one or two flakes of crushed garlic (*lasan*). Boil till they turn red. Filter. Use as ear drops.

❑ For pain due to boils, heat 1 teaspoon each of garlic (*lasan*) and carom seeds (*ajwain*) in 2 tablespoons gingelly oil (*til ka tel*) till they turn red in colour. Strain and cool. When cooled to body temperature, put some drops into the ears.

EAR INFECTION

Remedy (Nuskhe)...

❑ Extract 1 teaspoon juice from mango leaves. Slightly warm and use as ear drops when bearably hot.

EAR - PUS FORMATION INSIDE THE EARS

Remedy (Nuskhe)...

❑ In the case of pus inside the ears, warm 1 tbsp onion juice on fire and put 2-3 drops into the ears, 2-3 times a day. For onion juice, grate onion and squeeze well to take out the juice. Onion juice is also helpful in other types of ear problems.

❑ Pus formation inside the ears can be definitely cured by putting in a few drops of the juice obtained by crushing or grinding the flowers of bitter gourd (*karela*) plant.

ECZEMA

What is Eczema?

It is a skin infection.

Causes...

- Changes in temperature and humidity.
- Chemical irritants such as - pesticides, astringent, perfumes, harsh soaps, detergents and household cleaners.
- Allergies to dust, pollen etc.

Symptoms...

Bleeding on skin surface. Pus or other discharges, itchiness.

Remedy (Nuskhe)...

☐ Rub a nutmeg (*jaiphal*) against a smooth stone slab with a little water and make a paste. Apply on affected parts. (*Note*: It is believed by some rural, old practitioners that instead of water, one's own early morning saliva can be used for better results.)

☐ Add 1 teaspoon camphor (*kapoor*) to 1 teaspoon sandalwood paste and apply on the affected areas.

☐ Grind potatoes to a fine paste and thoroughly mix lemon juice into it and apply it to eczema, itches etc.

☐ Mix a paste of turmeric (*haldi*) and neem leaves (1:1) in a little gingelly oil (*til ka tel*) and apply on affected areas.

- Take ¼ cup juice extracted out of the leaves of bitter gourd *(karela)* plant, 2 tablespoons coconut oil *(naarial ka tel)*, ½ cup neem leaves and grind all these together. Apply it to the parts affected by eczema, itches etc. and they will be cured if you continue this treatment regularly for a few days.

- Eczema can be cured by regularly eating the kernel out of the seeds of melon *(kharbooje ki giri)* or even by regularly eating the melon fruit.

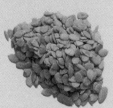

EPILEPSY

What is epilepsy?

A chronic neurological disorder that is characterized by recurrent unprovoked epileptic siezures or convulsions.

Triggers...

- Certain environmental factors can lead to an increased likelihood of seizures in someone with epilepsy.

- Tiredness and sleep deprivation.

- Constipation.

- Stress or anxiety, Physical trauma like going on a roller coaster.

Symptoms...

Sudden spasms of head, trunk and extremeties.

Remedy (Nuskhe)...

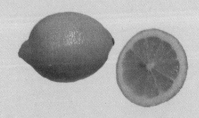

- Apply fresh lemon juice on the head. Massage well before showering off.

EYES

Eyes are one of the most sensitive parts of our body and can be afflicted by various problems. Splash tap water several times into the eyes when you daily wash your face in the mornings. This will help to maintain perfect eyesight up to ripe old age.

10 GOLDEN TIPS FOR HEALTHY EYES

1. Wash your eyes daily with cold water before going to bed.
2. Never look directly at the sun with naked eyes.
3. Avoid applying mascara to the eyes too fequently.
4. When you read, let the light fall on the book or paper from your left side.
5. Never read in dim or insufficient light.
6. Let the book or paper you read be about 15 inches from your eyes.
7. Do not read while traveling.
8. Frequently close and open your eyes while reading.
9. Do not wear spectacles which are cracked, scratched or dirty.
10. Using hair-dye will adversely affect the eyes. Use natural dyes like mehandi, for as long as possible.

EYES BURNING OR IRRITATION

❑ Grind an onion with 1 teaspoon each black pepper and poppy seeds (*khuskhus*) soaked in ½ cup milk. Apply this paste on the head. Allow it to dry for 15-20 minutes. Wash in warm water.

❑ Mix the juice of bottle gourd (*karela*) and sesame oil (*til ka tel*) in the ratio of 4:1, and heat till the moisture evaporates completely. Once cool, use it for massaging the head.

❑ For irritation of eyes, mix ¼ cup plain water with 1 tablespoon of rose-water (*gulab jal*) and wash eyes with it, 2-3 times a day.

EYES HAVING DARK CIRCLES AROUND THEM

❑ Take one teaspoon tomato juice, ½ teaspoon lemon juice, a pinch of turmeric (*haldi*) powder & a little gram flour (*besan*). Make a paste & apply. Leave for 10 minutes & wash off.

❑ Drink tomato juice with a few mint leaves a little lemon juice & salt.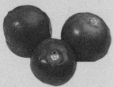

❑ Soak cotton wool in cucumber (*kheera*) or potato juice & apply around the eyes. You will find a change in 2-3 weeks.

FOR IMPROVING EYESIGHT, REMOVING GLASSES

❑ Mix seeds of cardamom (*chhoti ilaichi*) along with 1 tablespoon honey. Eat every day.

❑ 40 DAYS THERAPY - Mix equal quantities of almonds (*badaam*), cleaned fennel (*moti saunf*) and sugar candy *(mishri)*. Grind all together to a powder and store in a glass bottle. Every night before going to bed, drink 1 level tablespoon of this mixture mixed in 1 glass of milk. Continue for 40 days and see the result for yourself! For children reduce the quantity to half. Do not drink water for at least 2 hours after having this drink.

EYES-REMOVING FORIEGN PARTICLE

❑ Dissolve ¼ teaspoon of boric acid powder in ½ cup water and wash your eyes with it 2-3 times.

❑ Occasionally put in a drop of refined castor oil into your eyes to rid them of any dirt and to keep them clean and clear.

EYE STRAIN

❑ Any kind of work that causes eyestrain such as reading for long hours or working on computers can be relieved by focusing your eyes on a far away (distant) object for 2 minutes after every one hour.

❑ Nothing is more helpful when the eyes are tired than 10 minutes complete rest in a dark room. This relieves strain and relaxes muscles.

❑ "Palming" - An excellent way of resting the eyes. To do this, shut your eyes, not too lightly, but just so that the lids fall naturally and easily. Now cup your hands (palms), and place them gently over the closed eyes. Do it for a few moments during the day.

❑ Boil ½ teaspoon fennel seeds (saunf) in a cup of water till it is reduced to half. Cover and keep aside to cool. Strain through a fine strainer. Use as eye drops.

❑ Boil apple peel with water for a few minutes. Strain and sweeten with honey. Drink this or use it as an eye wash (for eye wash, honey can be omitted) for beneficial results in all eye problems

❑ From the early times our grandmothers have been recommending amla murabba for good eyes and health. It is also recommended for pregnant women. In both the above conditions, it does a world of good due to its high medicinal value.

❑ Mangoes are very rich in vitamin A and so their liberal consumption is very beneficial in various eye disorders. Night blindness, very common in undernourished children, is caused due to vitamin A deficiency. These patients benefit greatly by liberal consumption of mangoes.

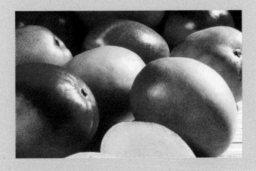

FAINTING

Remedy (Nuskhe)...

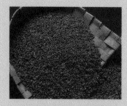

❏ A hot poultice of carom seeds (*ajwain*) may be used as dry fomentation for hands and feet.

FATIGUE

Causes...

Overworks, anaemia, past illness.

Symptoms...

Body pain, strong urge to rest or sleep.

Remedy (Nuskhe)...

❏ Take a glass of grapefruit with 1 tbsp of lemon juice to dispel fatigue and general tiredness after a day's work.

FEET

They are the most used part of the body and therefore prone to various problems. Should be very well looked after especially if diabetic.

FEET: CRACKED HEELS

- Mix equal quantities of glycerin and lemon juice. Apply every night before going to bed. This mixture can be made and stored in a glass bottle.

- Massage your feet with castor oil every night (in winters) for 2-3 minutes and then wear socks at night.

- Grind equal amounts of neem leaves & turmeric (*haldi*). Apply on affected area.

- Finely grind a handful of henna (*mehendi*) leaves. Add 2 tablespoons lemon juice and apply on the feet.

- Mix the juice of bottle gourd (*lauki*) and sesame oil (*til ka tel*) in the ratio 4:1 and heat till all the moisture has evaporated. Bottle and use over cracked skin

- Mix 1 cup bottle gourd *(lauki)* juice with ¼ cup sesame oil *(til ka tel)* and heat till the water evaporates. Massage regularly over chapped hands and heels. To take out juice, grate the lauki and squeeze through a muslin cloth to get juice.

- To heal cracked feet, wear one size larger slippers than your feet, when at home.

- Apply a paste of sandalwood powder mixed with desi ghee.

FEET-TIRED

- Bathe tired feet in a basin of hot water with 2 tablespoonfuls of salt or 2 tablespoons of vinegar *(sirka)* dissolved in it.

- Rub glycerine on tired feet at bed time and by next morning you will find them fresh and supple.

FOOT, ATHLETE'S

What is Athletes foot?

A fungal infection of the feet. Usually occurs between the toes.

Causes...

Condition easily spreads in public places such as communal showers, locker rooms and fitness centres.

Symptoms...

Itching, stinging and burning between your toes, soles of your feet. Itchy blisters, cracking and peeling skin between toes.

Remedy (Nuskhe)...

❑ Keeping your feet clean and dry is enough to discourage the growth of this fungal infection. Remember, it is infectious and you must keep and wash your shoes, socks and towel separately. To soothe the broken areas of your feet, simply soak them for 10 minutes in a footbath of apple cider vinegar mixed with water.

FOOT CORNS

Remedy (Nuskhe)...

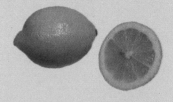

- ❑ Tie a fresh slice of lemon over the corn (painful area) and keep it all night.
- ❑ Massage castor oil for 2-3 minutes on the corns every morning and night before sleeping. In 3-4 weeks the corns will disappear.
- ❑ Mash 1-2 cloves (*laung*) & garlic (*lasan*) and tie over the corns. Leave overnight.
- ❑ To remove corns, massage the affected part with ice for 2-3 minutes. Rub turpentine oil on the corn and bandage it. In the morning the corn will come out. But continue to apply turpentine oil for the next few days.
- ❑ Vaseline rubbed on corns at night provides relief.

FEVER

What is fever?

Having fever means that your body temperature is higher than normal. Normal body temperature is 98.6° F.

Causes...

Something inside your body such as infection causes the temperature to go up. Fever is a natural phenomenon which the body adopts to indicate and fight illness.

Symptoms...

Increased body temperature, fatigue, body pain, dizziness, headache.

Remedy (Nuskhe)...

☐ Boil 1 tablespoon tulsi leaves with 1 teaspoon powdered cardamom (*chhoti illaichi*) in 2 teacups water. Take 1 cup of this decoction with milk and sugar to taste, 2 or 3 times a day.

☐ Tea made by boiling 1 teaspoon fenugreek seeds (*methi dana*), taken twice or thrice a day provides excellent remedy. (A little honey or lemon juice can be added).

☐ The neem leaf decoction taken with pepper powder lowers temperature.

☐ ½ teaspoon ground pepper is mixed in warm water along with 1 teaspoon palm candy (sugar obtained from palm). This drink is taken at bedtime.

☐ Apply sandalwood paste on the forehead to bring the temperature down.

☐ Sweet lime (*mousami*) or its juice is easily digested. It quenches thirst, is cooling and highly nourishing. An ideal food during sickness when other food is not permitted.

☐ Mix 1 teacup fresh lemon juice in tender coconut water and drink.

FLATULENCE

See gas problems on next page.

GAS PROBLEMS

What is Gas?

The presence of a mixture of gases known as flatus in the digestive tract. These are expelled from the rectum.

Causes

- Incomplete Digestion.
- Eating foods high in certain polysaccharides. These include beans, lentils, milk, onions, radish, sweet potatoes, cheese, cashews and cruciferous vegetables like cauliflower and broccoli.

Symptoms

Abdominal pain, bloating and belching (*dakaar*)

Remedy (Nuskhe)...

- ❑ Mix 1 tsp dhania powder with ¼ tsp mitha soda ¼ salt or ¼ tsp ajwain. Take twice daily.
- ❑ Chew slightly and swallow 2 flakes of garlic after meals along with a deseeded munakka. Very soon all the gas will be out.
- ❑ Eat 1 tsp coriander (*dhania*) powder (grind *dhania* seeds at home) with water after meals for a few days.
- ❑ Mix ¼ teaspoon dry ginger powder (*saunth*) with a pinch of asafoetida (*hing*) & a pinch of black salt (*kala namak*) in a little warm water and drink it.

- Mix 1-2 teaspoons brandy with warm water & drink for immediate relief from gas and stomach ache due to gas.

- Powder together dry ginger (*saunth*) with black pepper (*kali mirch*), equal amounts, say 1 teaspoon each along with 3-4 cardamom (*chhoti ilaichi*) seeds. Have ½ teaspoon of this mixed with water to relieve gas.

- Apply a paste of asafoetida (*hing*) mixed with water on the stomach.

- Make a coarse powder (*churan*) of equal amounts of cumin seeds (*jeera*), carom seeds (*ajwain*), black peppercorns (*sabut kali mirch*) and fenugreek seeds (*methi daana*). Have ½ teaspoon with water.

- To prevent gas from forming, chew a piece of fresh ginger after meals, regularly.

GOLDEN RULES FOR SUFFERING PATIENTS

- Avoid heavy (fried), spicy food. Do not eat very large meals, instead eat small meals every 2 hours.

- Do some exercise. Even a walk will do wonders.

GOUTY PAINS

What is Gout?

A painful form of arthritis which affects the big toe, but can also affect ankle, knee, foot, hand, elbow and wrist. Men are atleast 4 times more likely to develop gout than women.

Causes:

Excess uric acid in the body results in crystalline deposits in the joints which results in the joint inflammation.

Symptoms:

- Pain, swelling of the joint.
- Redness and tenderness of the joint area.

Remedy (Nuskhe)...

❏ Mix mustard oil and rectified alcohol (1 part oil to 40 parts alcohol) and use as a lotion.

❏ Make a poultice of ground fenugreek seeds (*methi dana*); use on the affected part.

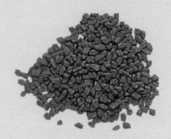

HAIR

Dadi maa says – if you take care of your hair, it will add to your looks and well being. Hair if neglected can break or fall, grey prematurely or be afflicted with dandruff. Common hair problems and remedies are given below –

DULL AND COARSE HAIR

Remedy (Nuskhe)...

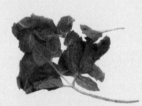

❑ Grind fresh fenugreek (*methi*) leaves to a paste and apply the leaf paste over the scalp before a bath.

HAIR FALLING AND LOSS

Remedy (Nuskhe)...

❑ Take a handful of neem leaves and boil them in 4 cups water. After cooling and filtering, use the decoction for rinsing hair.

❑ Mix equal quantities of dried curry leaves (*curry patta*), lime peel (*nimbu ka chhilka*), *shikakai*, fenugreek seeds (*methi daana*) & green gram (*moong sabut*) and grind them finely. Store and use as a substitute for soap or shampoo.

❑ Grind fenugreek (*methi*) seeds with some water and apply the paste on the head. Leave for at least 40 minutes before washing. Use every morning for a month.

❑ Apply a little almond oil (*badaam ka tel*) on scalp frequently and massage.

HAIR GREYING

Remedy (Nuskhe)...

- Wet a lemon half and rub lemon into the scalp well. Wash off after it turns dry.
- Grind 1 tablespoon each, pulp of amla and lemon juice. Massage this into the hair before going to bed. Wash it next morning.
- Soak shredded ginger (*adrak*) in honey. Eat a spoonful every morning.

HAIR THINNING

Remedy (Nuskhe)...

- Bathe the hair in 1 cup coconut milk twice or thrice a week for a few months.

HEADACHE, GENERAL

What is headache?

Pain in the head is called a headache.

Causes...

Poor eyesight, fatigue, cough, cold, fever and injury.

Symptoms...

It can be a throbbing pain between the eyes or pain in the head, sometimes nausea and dizziness.

Remedy (Nuskhe)...

- ❑ Peel and core a ripe apple. Eat with a little salt every morning on an empty stomach. Continue for a week. This yields good results even in case of chronic headaches.

- ❑ Roast some ajwain dry on a tawa. Tie it in a muslin bag and sniff frequently.

- ❑ Make a paste of 2-3 powdered cloves (*laung*) and salt. Apply this paste on the forehead.

- ❑ A paste made of dry ginger (*saunth*) with a little water or milk when applied to the forehead also gives relief.

- ❑ Mix 1 teaspoon finely ground cinnamon (*dalchini*) in 1 teaspoon water and apply on the forehead. It is very effective in headache due to exposure to cold air.

- ❑ Crush an onion and apply the paste on the head.

- ❑ Tulsi Tea: Mix 8-10 basil (*tulsi*) leaves, ½" piece ginger (*adrak*), 7 black pepper corns (*sabut kali mirch*) powdered coarsely in 1 large cup (200 ml) water. Boil for 2 minutes. Remove from heat, cover and keep for 2-3 minutes. Strain, add boiled milk, sugar and drink warm. Lie down covering yourself with a sheet for 5-10 minutes. It is very helpful in headaches, cold, indigestion. Drink 2-3 times a day. For children reduce quantity to half.

HEADACHE DUE TO EXPOSURE TO COLD AIR

Remedy (Nuskhe)...

❑ Mix 1 teaspoon finely ground cinnamon (*dalchini*) in 1 teaspoon water and apply on the affected parts.

❑ Follow the simple Chinese accupressure technique and say goodbye to those nasty headaches. This can be done anywhere and at any time. Place your thumb on the web of skin between the thumb and index finger of your other palm and apply pressure for about two minutes. Repeat on the other hand. However, this Chinese accupressure massage is not recommended for pregnant women.

HEADACHE ON ONE SIDE

Remedy (Nuskhe)...

❑ Mix 1 teaspoon each of the following powders and store: camphor (*kapoor*), nutmeg (*jaiphal*), cardamom (*chhoti ilaichi*) and cloves (*laung*). Take 2 pinches with warm water.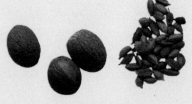

❑ Powder equal quantities of liquorice (*mulethi*) & cumin (*jeera*). Take ¼ teaspoon every day along with 1 teaspoon honey for a month.

❑ For half-head ache, grind together 1 onion and 3-4 peppercorns *(kali mirch)* in a little water, strain to get juice. Put a few drops juice in the nostril opposite to the side of head ache.

❑ Any kind of headache or even migraine can be relieved by ice packs. Place a few ice cubes in a polythene bag and apply this on the forehead and temples to ease the pain (avoid in winter).

❑ In case of headache mix 1 teaspoon dry ginger *(saunth)* with 2 tbsp water to a paste. Apply on the forehead to provide quick relief.

- Make a paste of 1" stick cinnamon *(dalchini)*, 4-5 peppercorns *(sabut kali mirch)*, ½" piece of ginger *(adrak)* and 4 teaspoons of powdered dried ginger *(saunth)*. Apply this thinly on the forehead. Rest and relax allowing it to dry. Then remove by washing it off.

HEAD HEAVINESS

Remedy (Nuskhe)...

- Grind the fresh amla fruit into a fine paste and apply on affected parts.
- Grind 2 to 3 cloves *(laung)* into a fine paste along with ½ teaspoon dried ginger *(saunth)* and apply on nose and forehead.

HEART PROBLEMS

The size of one's heart is usually the size of one's own fist and it weighs about 350-400 gms. It starts beating even before birth and continues to work without rest as long as we live. It beats 72 times per minute. Oxygen is carried by the blood through the coronary arteries which are the blood vessels supplying the heart.

The oxygen demand of the heart and the oxygen supply by the coronary arteries is always kept in balance in health. As the oxygen demand of the heart increases with exercise, emotion, eating etc. the oxygen supply also proportionately increases. When the oxygen demand and supply is not in balance, it results in heart attack. This is mainly due to the obstruction in the coronary arteries due to cholesterol which results in reduced blood supply to the heart.

In the initial stages, the heart trouble manifests as Angina Pectoris, that is severe central or left-sided chest pain. Later on, as the disease advances, it results in myocardial infarction – heart attack.

Patients must avoid ghee, butter, cheese, coconut oil, egg yolk, nuts, cream, organ meat (liver, brain). They can take greens, vegetables, onion, garlic, lean fish, white of the egg. As much as possible they should take boiled or steamed foods rather than fried food. For cooking gingelly (til) oil and sunflower oil can be used. Consume soya beans - they are excellent for the heart.

Symptoms of heart-attack

- Shortness of breath after slight exertion.
- Pain or tightness in the chest, often running down the left arm.
- Swelling in the ankles and abdomen.
- Dizziness, light-headedness, or vertigo.
- Seeing double (a particularly dangerous sign).
- Continuing indigestion.
- Persistent headache.
- Fatigue without valid reason.

Dadi maa recommends...

HEART PAIN

❑ Boil ½ teaspoon sandalwood powder in 1 cup water. Drink thrice daily.

HEART PALPITATION

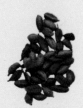

❑ Boil ¼ teaspoon powdered cardamom (*chhoti ilaichi*) seeds in thin tea water and drink.

HEART PROBLEM

❑ Eat ¼ teaspoon asafoetida (*hing*) along with one large raisin (*kishmish*) every day.

❑ Eat or swallow with water 1 or 2 cloves of peeled chopped or crushed garlic (*lasan*) 1st thing in the morning.

HEART WEAKNESS

❑ Regular intake of ripe bananas strengthens the heart.

❑ Apples are high in potassium and phosphorus content and very low (practically nil) in sodium. This fact is of great advantage in heart diseases.

❑ A weak heart benefits tremendously by the consumption of dates. Soak a few dates in water overnight. Crush them the next morning in the same water (remove seeds) and drink it at least 2-3 times a week for strengthening a weak heart.

❑ Grapes tone up the heart and are beneficial in cardiac pain and palpitations. The disease is controlled effectively if the patient goes on an exclusive grape diet for a few days.

- Orange juice sweetened with honey is a great nourishing and energy giving food. It is therefore recommended for heart patients particularly when one is on a liquid diet. It is also a good remedy against the thickening of arterial walls.

HEART BURN

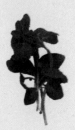

- Add 1 tablespoon mint (*pudina*) leaves to 1 cup water. Take twice or thrice a day.

HEAT STROKE

- Have the cooling drink '*panna*'. To prepare this, roast unripe or green mangoes in hot ashes. Extract the pulp and mix with water and sugar. You may even pressure cook the mangoes if you cannot make provision for the ashes.
- Eat raw onions with both the meals.
- Before you get out of the house drink a glass of butter milk or water.
- Apply some sandalwood oil on the forehead.

HEELS HAVING PAIN

Remedy (Nuskhe)...

- Mix equal amounts by weight of carom seeds (*ajwain*), onion seeds (*kalaunji*) fenugreek seeds (*methi daana*) and *sabut isabgol*. Have 1 tablespoon every day first thing in the morning. If you like you can grind them slightly in a blender — makes it more effective. This treatment takes a couple of months but is a sure shot remedy.

Note: *Sabut isabgol*, tiny very light pinkish particles, will be available with your grocer or if you request him he will get it for you from the wholesale market. Do not use the husk which is generally used by people for constipation as that is less effective but not harmful. If *sabut isabgol* is not available husk can be used but it takes longer for the pain to go.

HEPATITIS

What is Hepatitis?

It means liver inflammation. The inflammation makes the liver stop working well. This can lead to scarring called cirrhosis.

Causes...

Alcohol or certain drugs, it also happens after a viral infection.

Symptoms...

A short, mild flu like illness, nausea and vomitting, diarrhoea, loss of appetite, weight loss, jaundice, itchy skin

Remedy (Nuskhe)...

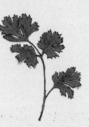

❑ 1 to 2 teaspoon fresh juice of coriander (*dhania*) leaves is mixed in 1 cup buttermilk and taken 2-3 times.

HICCUPS

Remedy (Nuskhe)...

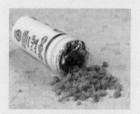

- ❑ Swallow ½ teaspoon mustard seeds (*sarson*) mixed with ½ teaspoon pure ghee.

- ❑ Drink ½ glass water, slowly.

- ❑ Keep a teaspoon of sugar in your mouth and suck slowly.

- ❑ Grind 4 green cardamom (*chhoti ilaichi*) well. Boil it in 2½ cups or ½ litre water. When about 1 cup water remains, remove from fire and sieve it through a muslin cloth. When warm, drink a glassful. Works like magic.

- ❑ Hold your breath as long as you can.

- ❑ Gargle with plain water, hot or cold, for at least a minute.

- ❑ Pull out your tongue.

- ❑ Suck 2-3 small pieces of fresh ginger (*adrak*). This helps in hiccups which keep re-occurring.

- ❑ Take asafoetida (*hing*) with little ghee.

INDIGESTION

A good digestive system is an indication of good health. Many diseases stem from poor digestive capacity. Health and ill health depends to a large extent on the power of digestion.

What is indigestion?

Our digetive system breaks up all that we eat or drink to useful components which the body requires to lead a healthy life. Any disturbance in this system leads to indigestion.

Causes...

- Eating too fast, especially by eating high-fat foods quickly
- Excessive acid accumulation in the stomach.
- Overconsumption of alcohol

Symptoms...

Frequent or loose bowel movements, gas, flatulance (feeling bloated), nausea, vomitting, dizziness, feeling feverish, acidity, burning sensation in stomach or chest.

Remedy (Nuskhe)...

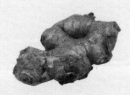

- ❑ Mix 1 teaspoon of ginger juice (*adrak ka rus*) and 1 teaspoon of lemon juice (*nimbu ka rus*). Open a bottle of soda into it. Salt or sugar can also be added according to taste.

- ❑ Put 2-3 tender leaves of tulsi in a glass of water overnight and drink this water early in the morning. This will clean your bowels and purify your blood.

- The simplest treatment for indigestion - eat ½ teaspoon carom seeds (ajwain).

- Have a glass of buttermilk (lassi) - churn together in a mixer, ½ cup curd, ½ teaspoon jeera (cumin seed), 4-5 curry leaves and 1" piece ginger chopped and ½ cup water.

- Roast 100 gm aniseed (saunf) on a griddle (tawa) till light brown. Cool and rub between palms to separate chaff. Grind it into powder. Mix the saunf powder with 100 gm cleaned carom seeds (ajwain) and 100 gm powdered sugar. Store in a bottle. A spoonful of this after meals benefits all those who suffer from indigestion and flatulence.

- Boil ½ tsp dry ginger powder (saunth) and ½ tsp jaggery (gur) in 1 cup water. Drink it warm two to three times a day.

- For indigestion, drink 1 cup hot water mixed with 2 teaspoons ginger juice and 1 teaspoon honey.

- Nausea, Acidity and Indigestion - Indigestion that is caused by overeating or some other cause can be cured by sucking 1-2 black cardamoms (badi ilaichi) with a little sugar.

- Boil 5-6 sticks of powdered cinnamon (dalchini) in a glass of water. Add a pinch of pepper powder and little honey. A tablespoon of the above concoction taken ½ hour after meals relieves indigestion and flatulence (gas).

- Mix ¼ teaspoon pepper powder, ¼ teaspoon of cumin (jeera) powder is a glass of buttermilk. Have this 1-2 times a day.

- Chew your food well and do not eat bellyful. Consume slightly less than your appetite.

- Add 1 teaspoon fresh grated ginger (adrak) to 1 cup water. Cover and simmer on low heat for 5 minutes. Strain and drink 1-2 times a day.

- Soak one teaspoon of celery seeds in a glass of buttermilk for 5-6 hours. Grind in the same buttermilk and drink it 1-2 times a day.

- Grapes form a light food and so help in overcoming indigestion. They have a soothing effect on excessive secretion of bile and the burning sensation in the stomach.

- Eat 1 tsp dhania powder with a little water after meals for few days.

INSECT BITES

Remedy (Nuskhe)...

❑ Drink 2 to 3 teaspoons coriander (*dhania*) leaf juice mixed in 1 cup water. Also apply sandalwood paste on the affected area.

❑ Take 1 teaspoon basil (*tulsi*) leaf juice and drink with water. Also apply externally.

INSOMNIA (SLEEPLESSNESS)

What is insomnia?

Inability to sleep is called insomnia. If a person is unable to sleep for days it can lead to death. Sleep is an essential requirement as it restores energy and permits us to lead a healthy life.

Causes...

Execessive fatigue, Post illness, Stress.

Remedy (Nuskhe)...

❑ Avoid drugs. Try a cup of hot milk at bed time after a warm bath.

❑ If you do not fall asleep after going to bed try the following method: Lie on your back and do deep breathing for about 15 times and then lie on the side. You will easily go to sleep.

❑ Sometimes you can be so tired you can't even go to sleep! Try taking a hot and then a cold bath. It will refresh you.

❑ It is said that raw onion eaten daily induces sound sleep.

❑ Add 2 teaspoons of honey to a big cupful of water and have it before going to bed. Babies generally fall asleep after having honey.

- A cup of warm milk sweetened with honey should be taken before going to bed. Have it everyday.

- Juice of celery leaves (*ajwain ka patta*) with thick ribs & brittle stalks mixed with a tablespoon of honey when had at night before retiring helps to relax into a restful sleep.

- Fry cumin seeds (*jeera*) in a little ghee & grind to a powder. A teaspoon of this mixed with the pulp of a ripe banana should be taken at night regularly.

- 2 teaspoons juice of fenugreek (*methi*) leaves along with 1 teaspoon honey may be taken daily.

- Soak 1 tablespoon leaves of fresh mint (*pudina*) in 1 cup water for 30 minutes. Drink every night. (Do not boil.)

- Take seeds of watermelon and white poppy seeds (*khuskhus*) and grind them separately. Mix equal amounts by weight. Have 3/4 teaspoon once in the morning and once before sleeping. Take for 1-3 weeks as needed.

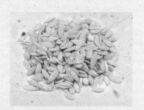 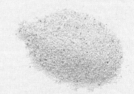

INTESTINAL WORMS

Remedy (Nuskhe)...

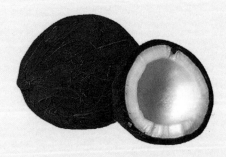

☐ Eat papayas frequently.

☐ Take 5-10 seeds of bitter gourd (*karela*) and crush them. Fry them in a little *ghee*. Take twice daily.

☐ For 3-5 year old children - Give a tiny piece of jaggery (*gur*), about 10 gm, first thing in the morning to the child. Let the child rest for 15 minutes. Now give ¼ teaspoon of ground carom seeds *(ajwain)* with a glass of water. (Grind ajwain and store in an air tight bottle). For adults you may increase the quantity to double.

☐ Fry 1 teaspoon dried neem flowers in 1 teaspoon *ghee* and mix with 1 cup boiled rice and eat twice or thrice a day.

☐ Slice and dry the kernel of mango pit (*guthli*) and mango powder along with 1 tbsp fenugreek seeds (*methi daana*). Take 1 teaspoon mixed with buttermilk.

☐ Intestinal disorders or disturbances benefit a lot from the nicotinic acid content of dates. Hence liberal use of dates in your daily diet helps and encourages the growth of friendly bacteria in the intestines and cures intestinal disorders.

☐ Kernel of a ripe coconut is excellent for the expulsion of worms particularly tapeworm. Grate the coconut and have 2 tablespoon of this followed by a dose of castor oil after 2-3 hours. Repeat this everyday till the worms have been expelled.

INFLAMMATION OF THE GUMS (PYORRHOEA)

What is inflamation of the gums?

Swollen and/or bleeding gums.

Causes...

Poor dental hygeine, infection.

Symptoms...

Pain in the gums, swelling, bleeding.

Remedy (Nuskhe)...

❑ Pyorrhoea can be cured by eating oranges *(santra)* daily and rubbing the gums with their skins.

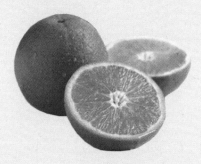

INFLAMMATION OF SPLEEN

What is inflammation of spleen?

Enlargement of the spleen. The spleen is located in the upper left part of the abdomen.

Causes...

Caused by certain diseases like malaria, leukemia, pernicious anaemia.

Symptoms...

The spleen destroys old blood cells, so when it gets enlarged the blood count is disturbed.

Remedy (Nuskhe)...

❑ In this condition, consumption of 2-3 figs along with a cup of curd at least twice a day is very beneficial. This should be continued for a few weeks.

❑ Liver and Spleen inflammation: Take a large slice of papaya with 1 teaspoon of honey every day to control the inflammation of spleen and liver. Avoid fats, starches, sugar, alcohol and tobacco.

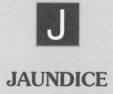

JAUNDICE

What is Jaundice?

Jaundice can be broadly classified as **infective** and **obstructive** jaundice.

A virus called **Hepatitis A**, is a common cause of infective jaundice. This virus is transmitted through water and food. Children are often affected.

The other viruses such as **Hepatitis B and Hepatitis C viruses** are transmitted through blood.

Causes...

Stones or growths, blocking the pathway of bile, contaminated food and water, liver malfunction, certain diseases, certain medicines, viruses, alcohol, certain vitamin deficiency.

Symptoms...

Yellow complexion, nausea, fatigue, itching, confusion, slow pulse, yellow eyes.

Remedy (Nuskhe)...

❑ Mash a ripe banana along with 1 tablespoon honey and eat twice a day for a few days.

❑ Frequently drink lemon juice.

❑ Take ¼ teaspoon turmeric (*haldi*) along with a glass of hot water 2 or 3 times daily.

- ½ teaspoon ginger juice with 1 teaspoon each fresh lime and mint (*pudina*) juice mixed with a tablespoon of honey, taken frequently.

- Finely grind some bel leaves. Take 1 teaspoon of this paste along with a pinch of black pepper and follow it with 1 cup of buttermilk thrice a day.

- A fine paste of tender papaya leaves, about ½ teaspoon paste, is taken with some water.

- Make a fine powder of 1 teaspoon each of crushed liquorice (*mulethi*) root, chicory seeds (*kaasni*) and rock salt (*kala namak*). Take ½ teaspoon with water twice daily.

- Wash 3-4 tender leaves of peepal tree. Grind the leaves to a paste with a little sugar or mishri. Mix the paste in 1 glass of water and then strain through a fine cloth, Have it twice a day for 3-7 days.

- Take a glass of butter milk (*lassi*) with a pinch of black pepper (*kali mirch*).

- Mix 1 teaspoon of glucose powder in a cup of water. Have it 3 times a day - morning, afternoon and night.

- Have juice of poodina with a little sugar early morning.

- Musk melon (*kharbooza*) is good for people suffering from jaundice as the toxins are removed through the urine by consuming this high water content fruit.

- Plums are beneficial for jaundice patients.

- Sugarcane juice (*ganne ka ras*).

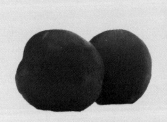
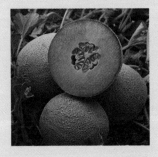
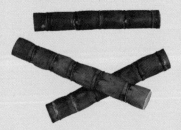

KIDNEY PROBLEMS

What is kidney problem?

The two kidneys - right and left in the body act like a filter and separate body wastes into urine, which is then flushed out through the urinary tract. If the kidneys fail to function properly - they can lead to grave problems.

Causes...

Could be congenital or acquired.

Symptoms...

Obstruction of flow of urine and pain.

Remedy (Nuskhe)...

❑ Frequent intake of coriander (*dhania*) tea: Boil or steep 2 tsp finely ground coriander (*dhania*) seeds in a glass of boiling hot water. Add sugar and milk to taste.

❑ Add more almonds to the daily diet.

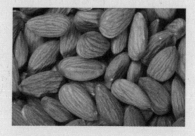

KIDNEY AND BLADDER STONES

Remedy (Nuskhe)...

☐ *Kulthi, which is like daal,* is the best remedy for stones.

Soak 250 gm *kulthi* in 3 litres (12 cups) water overnight. Next morning, boil it on low heat for 4 hours till about 1 litre (4 cups) water remains. Temper the dal water with 3-4 tbsp pure ghee. To temper (*chhownk*), heat ghee and add jeera and black pepper (*kali mirch*). Add some rock salt (*sendha namak*) and *haldi* too. Add tempered ghee to the dal soup. Have only this for lunch for 1-2 weeks. Drink as much as you can, atleast have 1 large cup of the soup every day as lunch. You may have 1 chapati with it if you cannot stay without roti. You may cook this daal like any other dal and eat with roti too but the above method of taking it as soup is still better.

☐ People suffering from these disorders benefit greatly by including almonds in their daily diets.

☐ Fig consumption is beneficial in these conditions. Boil 6-7 figs in 1 cup of water. Cool and drink daily for at least a month. In case of kidney stones drinking juice of fresh figs frequently is also very beneficial.

☐ Grind walnut kernels to a powder. Have 1 teaspoon of walnut powder, morning and evening to get rid of stones through the urine.

☐ Having cucumber (*kheera*) is very beneficial. Eat cucumber in the evenings. Avoid rice and spinach (*paalak*).

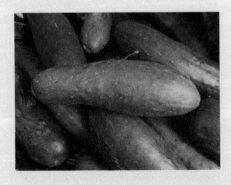

LACTATION IN MOTHERS

Dadi maa recommends...

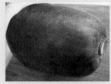

- *Breast feeding helps the womb to shrink back to its normal size more quickly.*

- Frequently, cook raw papayas (*kacha papita*) and eat.

- ½ teaspoon finely ground cinnamon (*dalchini*) taken every night along with 1 cup milk.

- A pinch of powdered cinnamon *(dalchini)* mixed with a little honey should be taken every night. It not only increases secretion of breast milk, but also checks early release of ova after child birth, delays occurrence of menstruation and prevents early conception.

- Mix together 1 teaspoon each cumin (*jeera*) powder & sugar and take with warm milk after dinner every day for a few days.

- Boil 2 teaspoons cumin (*jeera*) seeds in ½ cup water. Filter. Mix in ½ cup milk and 1 teaspoon honey. Drink once a day for a few days.

- Boil 2 teaspoons fennel seeds (*saunf*) in barley water and take twice or thrice a day.

- Grind a handful of bitter gourd (*karela*) leaves into a fine paste and apply on breasts.

- Grind together ½ cup cumin seeds (*jeera*), ½ cup aniseeds (*saunf*) and ½ cup sugar candy *(mishri)* to a powder. Have 1 teaspoon of it with milk, three times a day.

- A khichri like mixture prepared from roasted fenugreek seeds *(bhuna methi daana),* milk and sugar is given to increase breast milk.

LACTATION - STOPPING

- Tie warmed leaves of dhatura on the breasts.

LEGS, SWELLING AND PAIN

Remedy (Nuskhe)...

❑ Mix equal quantities of castor oil and lemon juice. Massage the affected area with this mixture. Also drink 1 cup warm water mixed with lemon juice and honey.

LICE

Remedy (Nuskhe)...

❑ Grind the seeds of neem into a fine powder and mix in some groundnut oil. Apply to the scalp. Allow it to remain overnight. Wash off next morning.

❑ Mix 1 teaspoon lemon juice with 1 teaspoon garlic (*lasan*) paste and apply on the head.

❑ Grind 7 to 8 almond (*badam*) kernels with 1 to 2 teaspoons lemon juice and apply on the hair.

LONGEVITY

Dadi maa recommends...

❑ 5 to 10 basil (*tulsi*) leaves taken along with water every morning on an empty stomach continuously for 108 days.

❑ ¼ to ½ teaspoon peeled and finely chopped ginger sprinkled with a pinch of rock salt (*sendha namak*) taken ½ hour before meals for 8-10 days will prove beneficial.

LIVER COMPLAINTS

Remedy (Nuskhe)...

- ❏ Have 2 tbsp juice of fresh amla, three times a day for 15-20 days. In case fresh amlas are not available, take 1 tsp of ground dried amlas with a little water.

- ❏ Frequently drinking pineapple juice is good for liver complaints.

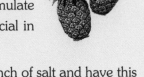

- ❏ When *jamuns* are in season, eat 200-300 gm on an empty stomach every day. Consumption of ripe jamuns is said to stimulate the liver. Very good for a weak liver.

- ❏ The malic, citric and tartaric acids found in grapes stimulate the liver and bile secretion. They are therefore beneficial in all liver disorders.

- ❏ Squeeze juice of ½ lemon in half glass water. Add a pinch of salt and have this three times a day.

LISPING, DEFECTIVE SPEECH (TUTLANA)

Remedy (Nuskhe)...

- ❏ Children should be given 1 fresh green amla to chew everyday for a few days. This will help in making the speech clear.

- ❏ Crush 7 blanched almonds *(badam giri)* and 7 black peppercorns *(saboot kali mirch)* with a few drops of water to a paste. Mix some powdered sugar candy *(mishri)* with it. Give it to the child on an empty stomach for a few days.

LEUCODERMA (WHITE PATCHES)

What is leucoderma?

Leucoderma, also called Vitiligo, in which depigmentation (white patches) of the skin occurs. It is by and large, of unknown actiology in the majority of cases.

Remedy (Nuskhe)...

❑ Seeds of psoralea (*babchi*) combined with seeds of tamarind (*imli*) are beneficial. Soak equal quantities of both the seeds in water for 3-4 days. Then shell and dry them in the shade. Grind into a paste and apply on the white patches for a week. If the application of this paste causes itching or the white spots become red and a fluid begins to ooze out, it should be discontinued. If there is no itching or reddening, babchi seeds should be taken internally also for 40 days.

❑ Another useful treatment for leucoderma is a red clay found by the riverside or on hill slopes. The clay should be mixed in ginger (*adrak*) juice and applied over the white spots once a day. The copper content in the clay seems to bring back skin pigmentation and ginger (*adrak*) juice serves as a mild stimultant, facilitating increased blood supply to the spots. Drinking water kept overnight in a copper vessel will also help.

❑ Burn a few dry dates (*chhuara*) along with the seeds into ash and powder them. Apply this ash mixed with *neem oil* once a day for two months.

❑ The patient should avoid tea, coffee, alcoholic beverages, all condiments, and highly flavoured dishes, pickles, sugar, white flour products, processed cereals like polished rice, pearl barley and tinned or bottled foods.

MOUTH AND TONGUE WOUNDS

Remedy (Nuskhe)...

❑ A tongue burnt by a hot eatable or a beverage can be really painful. You can cool the tongue by sucking a spoonful of sugar.

❑ In case of wounds inside the mouth & on the tongue, mix coriander (*dhania*) powder with a little honey. Eat it little by little.

❑ Eating leaves of tulsi will cure wounds inside the mouth, on the tongue and on the lips.

MOUTH ULCERS (*CHHALE*)

Remedy (Nuskhe)...

❑ Grind 1 small harad to a powder and apply on the chhala.

❑ Chew a small harad at night after dinner.

❑ Chew 4-5 tulsi leaves every morning and evening and take 2 sips of water after that. Eat for a week.

❑ Mix ¼ teaspoon of borax powder with 1 tablespoon glycerine and apply on the chhalas.

❑ Blisters in the mouth can be effectively treated by applying boro-glycerine or by gargling with a solution of potassium permanganate, the latter producing better results.

❑ Mix some coconut milk with honey and massage the gums 3 to 4 times a day.

❑ Gargle with (or apply) freshly extracted coconut milk from a ripe coconut frequently.

- Mix the pulp of a ripe bel fruit with jaggery (*gur*) and eat once a day.

- Prepare coriander (*dhania*) decoction by boiling 1 teaspoon coriander seeds (*sabut dhania*) in 1 cup water. Strain water & gargle frequently, when lukewarm.

- Chew one or two tender leaves of fig (*anjeer*) and leaf buds frequently and wash the mouth with warm water.

- Soak 1 tablespoon crushed liquorice (*mulethi*) root in 2 cups water for 2 to 3 hours and use it for gargling frequently.

- Boil 2 tablespoons fenugreek (*methi*) leaves along with ½ cup green gram (*sabut moong dal*) and 10 small onions. Eat regularly.

- Fenugreek seeds (*methi dana*), fried and powdered, to be added to drinking water. Drink 2-3 times daily for 2-3 days.

- Pour boiling water over fenugreek (*methi*) leaves. Keep aside till lukewarm. Strain and gargle with this infusion, 5-6 times daily for a couple of days.

- The sherbet of mulberry fruit (shahtoot) is very beneficial for people having ulcers (*chhale*) in the mouth and throat.

MEMORY IMPROVEMENT

- Take a mixture of 1 teaspoon honey and a pinch of finely powdered cinnamon (*dalchini*) every night regularly.

- Take ½ teaspoon black cumin (*kala jeera*) powder and mix it with honey. Eat small quantities of it twice a day.

- Memory can be improved if you make a habit of daily drinking 2 glasses of water before going to bed.

- Mix 1 teaspoon each amla root powder and white sesame seed (*safed til*) powder. Add 1 teaspoon honey and eat every day for a few days.

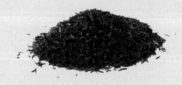

MENSTRUATION

Although menstruation is a natural phenomenon in women, they can be painful, delayed, excessive or irregular. Remedies for these conditions are listed below.

MENSTRUAL PAINS

❑ Boil 1 teaspoon saffron (*kesar*) in ½ cup water. Let it reduce to become 1 tablespoon. Divide this decoction into three portions and take with equal quantities of water, thrice daily for a couple of days.

❑ Grind a small piece of ginger (*adrak*), 1 flake garlic (*lasan*) and a few leaves of drumstick (*sahijan*), if available, to a paste with a little salt and water. Take about two tablespoon on an empty stomach in the morning and before going to bed on the first three days of the period. Repeat this treatment for 3 months.

❑ Add a handful of common salt to your bath water to get relief from painful menstruation.

❑ Mix 1 ripe banana with a little amla powder, honey and sugar and eat it daily for a few days. This is good for all menstrual complaints and also white discharge.

MENSTRUATION DELAYED

Remedy (Nuskhe)...

❑ Take ½ teaspoon finely ground cinnamon (*dalchini*) every night along with 1 cup milk.

❑ Powder 1 teaspoon dried mint (*pudina*) leaves and take with 1 teaspoon honey, thrice daily.

❑ 6 to 8 almonds, crushed and mixed in 1 cup milk along with 1 egg yolk, ½ teaspoon sesame (*til*) powder and 1 teaspoon honey. Take once or twice a day.

MENSTRUATION, EXCESSIVE BLEEDING

Remedy (Nuskhe)...

- Grind some bel leaves into a fine paste. Take 1 teaspoon with warm water and drink some cold water as well.

- Grind 10 fresh buds of figs (*anjeer*) and apply on the lower abdomen below the navel for a few hours. Repeat this frequently.

- Boil 1 teaspoon coriander (*dhania*) seeds in 2 cups water till it is reduced to 1 cup. Add sugar to taste and drink when lukewarm. Repeat twice or thrice a day.

- In the case of excessive flow during menstruation, get a few small and tender brinjals *(baingan)* fresh from the plant, grind them with a little water, squeeze out the juice, strain and drink it for 3 consecutive days before the commencement of the monthly period.

- If hibiscus flowers (China Rose) are ground to a pulp and mixed in a cup of milk and drunk, excessive menstrual flow ceases.

- Take 1 flake of garlic (*lasan*), a few neem (*margosa*) leaves and a small piece of turmeric (*haldi*). Grind them together to a fine paste and prepare small tablets and store. Eat one tablet per day for 3 days immediately preceding the commencement of the periods to cease excessive menstrual flow

- Take 1 teaspoon sugar and 2 teaspoon honey, mix them together and eat it daily for 5 days.

MENSTRUATION, PAINFUL AND IRREGULAR

- A piece of fresh ginger (*adrak*), ground and boiled in a cup of water. The infusion is taken thrice daily after meals along with sugar.

MORNING SICKNESS

Many women suffer from nausea and vomitting in the early months of pregnancy. Nausea is maximum in the mornings and hence it has been described as morning sickness. It usually ceases after the first three months, but may persist a little longer in some cases.

Remedy (Nuskhe)...

❑ One of the easiest ways to prevent morning sickness is to eat something before getting out of bed. A cup of tea with some biscuits or a piece of fruit eaten on waking up helps a lot.

❑ Mix 1 teaspoon each of fresh juice of mint (*pudina*) & lime along with 1 tablespoon honey. Take 3 times a day.

❑ Mix juice of 15-20 tender curry leaves (*curry patta*) with 2 teaspoon lemon juice and 1 teaspoon sugar. Take in the morning.

❑ Mix 1/8 teaspoon nutmeg (*jaiphal*) powder with 1 tablespoon freshly extracted amla juice. Take 3 times a day.

❑ ½ teaspoon ginger (*adrak*) juice with 1 teaspoon each fresh lime and mint (*pudina*) juice mixed with a tablespoon of honey, taken frequently.

MOSQUITO BITE

❑ Apply lemon juice diluted with water on body.

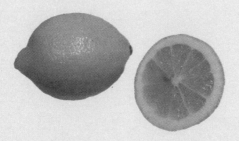

MOUTH INFECTION

❑ Powder dried mint (*pudina*). Use as toothpowder.

MOUTH INFLAMMATION

❑ Soak 1 tablespoon crushed liquorice (*mulethi*) root in 2 cups of water for 2 to 3 hours and use it for gargling frequently.

MOUTH ODOUR

❑ Tea made by boiling 1 teaspoon fenugreek seeds (*methi dana*), taken twice or thrice a day. A little honey or lemon juice can be added to improve the flavour.

MALARIA AND FEVERISH COLDS

❑ Consumption of grapefruit during feverish colds and Malaria is highly recommended. Grapefruit contains a natural 'quinine' which makes it very useful in malaria treatment. Boil half a grapefruit with some water and strain the pulp. Have this 1-2 times a day.

MIGRAINE

❑ Having grape juice in small quantities frequently (a few times daily) brings relief in migraine cases.

NOSE-RUNNING OR BLOCKED CONGESTION

❑ Before going to bed chew 7 peppercorns (*sabut kali mirch*) and 1 teaspoon sugar candy (*mishri*).

❑ Tulsi tea - When making tea, add 2 cloves (*laung*), 1 green cardamom (*chhoti ilaichi*), ½ teaspoon dried ginger powder (*saunth*) and 6 basil (*tulsi*) leaves, while boiling the water.

❑ Boil 7 peppercorns (*sabut kali mirch*) and 7 *batashas* in 1 cup water till ¼ cup water is left. Drink it hot and cover your head and body properly and rest for 10 minutes. Have it twice a day - once on empty stomach in the morning and once at night just before going to bed, for 2-3 days. If you have fever with the cold, add 7 leaves of tulsi also.

❑ Rub a nutmeg (*jaiphal*) on a smooth grinding stone along with some cow's milk. Apply this paste on forehead and nose.

❑ Crush a fistful of carom seeds (*ajwain*) and tie up in a cotton napkin and place it near the pillow.

❑ Put 1 teaspoon cardamom (*chhoti ilaichi*) seeds on burning coal and inhale the smoke.

❑ Make into a very fine powder equal quantities of the following: green cardamom (*chhoti ilaichi*) seeds, cinnamon (*dalchini*), black pepper (*kali mirch*) and cumin (*jeera*). Sniff this powder frequently to induce sneezing.

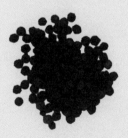
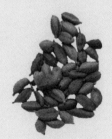
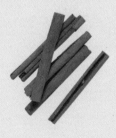

NOSE BLEEDING

What is nose bleed?

Nose bleed is a common problem that can be treated at home. Medically, it is known as epistaxis.

Causes...

Cold or flu, Allergies, Nasal tumor, Nose injury, Nose picking, Nasal infection.

Symptoms...

Expelling of blood from the nostrils.

Remedy (Nuskhe)...

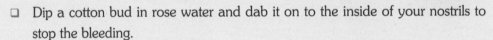

- ❏ Drop lemon juice in nostrils.
- ❏ Use juice of fresh coriander leaves (*dhania*) as nasal drops.
- ❏ Dip a cotton bud in rose water and dab it on to the inside of your nostrils to stop the bleeding.
- ❏ Mix ½ teaspoon borax (*suhaaga*) with a little water and apply the paste on both the nostrils. Bleeding stops instantly.
- ❏ If you put a stream of cold water on the head, bleeding from the nose usually stops.
- ❏ Excessive bleeding of the nose can be stopped by placing a piece of newspaper over the nose.
- ❏ For bleeding from the nose, drop the juice of pomegranate (*anar*) flowers into the nose.

OBESITY

❑ Mix lemon juice with honey and water. Drink a glass of this every morning.

❑ Mix 3 teaspoons lemon juice, ¼ teaspoon powdered black pepper (*kali mirch*) and 1 teaspoon honey in 1 cup water. Drink for 3 months.

❑ Eat 10 fresh, fully grown curry leaves (*curry patta*) every morning for 3 to 4 months.

❑ Eat a tomato before breakfast.

OLD AGE PROBLEMS (GENERAL DEBILITY)

❑ Boil 1 teaspoon ginger (*adrak*) in 1 cup water till reduced to ½ cup. Add to it ½ cup cow's milk, 2 green cardamoms (*chhoti ilaichi*), 5 strands of saffron (*kesar*) and 1 teaspoon sugar. Drink every morning.

P

PALMS, BURNING SENSATION

- ❑ Grind a handful of bitter gourd (*karela*) leaves into a smooth paste and apply on the affected areas of feet and palms frequently.

PHYSICAL WEAKNESS

- ❑ Soak 2 or 3 dried figs (*anjeer*) overnight in 1 cup water. Eat them along with 1 tablespoon honey the next morning. Continue for a month.

- ❑ Fry in 1 tablespoon butter, 2 teaspoons each of wheat flour, almond paste and poppy seeds (*khuskhus*) paste. Eat this along with 1 cup boiled fenugreek (*methi*) leaves.

PILES

What is piles?

Piles or haemorrhoids are very common. It is a thickening and inflammation of veins, inside or just outside the rectum. In external piles, there is a lot of pain, but not much bleeding. In the case of internal piles, there is discharge of dark blood. In some cases the veins burst and this results in what is known as bleeding piles.

Causes...

Chronic constipation and other bowel disorders, prolonged periods of standing or sitting, strenuous work, obesity, general weakness of the tissues of the body, mental tension, and heredity.

Symptoms...

Pain while passing stools, slight bleeding in the case of internal trouble, and feeling of soreness and irritation after passing a stool are the usual symptoms of piles. Itching, discomfort around the rectal area.

Remedy (Nuskhe)...

Precaution: Constipation should be avoided as it leads to an aggravation of piles.

❑ Mix 1 teaspoon fresh juice of mint (*pudina*) leaves with 1 teaspoon lemon juice & 1 tablespoon honey. Take 3 times a day.

❑ Boil a mashed ripe banana in 1 cup of milk & take 2-3 times a day.

❑ Mix juice of 15-20 tender curry leaves (*curry patta*) with 1 teaspoon honey & drink everyday.

❑ Take 1 tablespoon black cumin seeds (*kala jeera*) and roast them. Mix in another tablespoon of black cumin seeds (unroasted) and powder them finely. Take ½ teaspoon of this powder with a glass of water everyday.

❑ 3 teaspoon of the juice of the leaves of bitter gourd (*karela*) mixed with a glassful of buttermilk taken every morning for a month is a good remedy for piles.

❑ The juice of radish (*mooli*) or consuming fresh radish is very effective. The juice should be given in doses of 60-90 ml (¼-½ cup), morning & evening.

❑ Take ½ teaspoon each of dried and powdered pomegranate (*anaar*) flowers, poppy seeds (*khus khus*) & dried and powdered neem leaves, twice a day with milk for bleeding piles.

❑ Grind 1 onion to a paste. Mix with curd (*dahi*) and eat it once or twice a day for 7 days. Eating raw onion is very good.

❑ Have a glass of butter milk (*lassi*) every day after lunch. To 1 glass of *lassi* add ¼ tsp ground carom seeds (*pisi ajwain*) and a pinch of rock salt (*sendha namak*).

❑ Take equal quantities each of garlic (*lasan*), neem seed, asafoetida (*hing*) and dry ginger (*sukhi adrak*). Grind them all together with a little water. Make ¼ inch size tablets, dry them in shade and store them. Take 1-2 tablets morning and evening together with water for a few days.

- Finely powder the husk or the covering of the tamarind seed *(imli ka beej)*. Eat a pinch thrice daily for a week to cure bleeding piles.

- Dry the leaves of "touch me not" plant (*Mimosa pudica*) in shade and powder them. Add a teaspoonful of this powder to 1 cup of hot milk and have it at bed time. It is an excellent cure for piles.

- Extract 2 tbsp juice of bitter gourd *(karela)* and mix 1 tbsp of sugar candy *(mishri)* and drink first thing in the morning for 7 days. Wash and grate the *karela* and squeeze out the juice.

- For itching of anus, apply plain vaseline with boric powder or plain coconut oil *(narial ka tel)*. Pulp of tender coconut is used for piles and the oil from the nut when externally applied controls the pain due to piles.

- Figs being laxative in nature are a great help and an excellent remedy for piles. Clean 3-4 dried figs well. Wash with warm water and then soak them in 1 cup or 1 glass of water, preferably in an enamel container overnight. Next morning eat these and drink the water also in which they are soaked. Similarly soak 3-4 figs in the morning and have them in the evening. Continue this treatment for at least a month. As there is no straining at the time of evacuation, piles get cured in due course.

- Eating a few jamuns every morning either with salt or honey proves to be very effective in controlling and curing bleeding piles.

PIMPLES/ACNE/BLACKHEADS

Remedy (Nuskhe)...

- Application of fresh mint *(pudina)* juice over face every night cures pimples. Clean face with rose water *(gulab jal)* 2-3 times a day.

- The orange peel (*santare ka chilka*) is very valuable in the treatment of pimples too. Pound the peel with water on a piece of stone and apply on the affected area. When oranges are not in season, dry peels in the shade. Powder the dried peels. Sift to get a fine powder & store.

PRICKLY HEAT

Remedy (Nuskhe)...

❑ Mix 1 tablespoon sandalwood powder in some rose water to get a thin paste. Apply the paste on the affected parts. Wash off after ½ hour. Sandalwood powder is easily available in most cosmetic shops.

❑ For prickly heat on the shoulders and back of children, dip a piece of cotton in rose water (*gulab jal*) and dab it over the child's body. Repeat it twice a day and see the result.

❑ Mix ground cumin seeds (*jeera powder*) with coconut oil (*narial ka tel*) to get a thick solution. Apply on the body. Bathe it off after some time. Repeat this for few days or until cured.

❑ Apply rice water obtained by washing rice before cooking.

PAIN IN HIPS

Remedy (Nuskhe)...

❑ Extract some coconut milk from a ripe coconut. Cook some fenugreek (*methi*) leaves in it. Add an egg to it. Eat this 2-3 times a day for relief from pain in the hips.

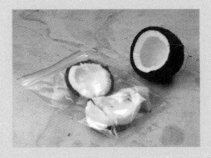

REPRODUCTIVE WEAKNESS

Remedy (Nuskhe)...

❑ Boil 1 cup milk with ½ teaspoon pepper powder and 6 to 8 crushed almonds. Take at bedtime.

RHEUMATIC PAIN

What is rheumatism?

The word rheumatism is derived from the Greek word 'rheuma', which means a swelling.

Causes...

Presence of toxic waste products in the blood caused by: too much meat in the diet, refined products, sugar, medical reasons, cold water. Concentrated toxic waste, settles around the joints and bone structure forming the basis of rheumatism.

Symptoms...

Fever, intense soreness, swelling and severe pain of the muscles, ligaments, tendons, or the joints.

Remedy (Nuskhe)...

❑ Boil 3 tablespoon powdered nutmeg (*jaiphal*) in 1 cup sesame oil (*til ka tel*). Cool and apply on affected parts.

❑ 2 to 3 teaspoons pepper powder is fried in 2 teaspoons sesame oil (*til ka tel*) until charred. When it is warm, apply on the affected areas and massage lightly.

❑ A 3-inch piece of dried ginger (*saunth*) to be ground with a grape-sized piece of asafoetida (*hing*) in milk. The paste to be applied on the affected area. The area should be exposed to the sun for imparting warmth.

RABIES

What is rabies?

The bite of a rabid (mad) dog results in rabies, which is fatal.

Symptoms...

The patient froths from the mouth and looses his mental balance.

Remedy (Nuskhe)...

❑ Remove the kernels out of the seeds of the bitter sponge gourd (*karela*), chop them fine and mix them with about ¼ litre of water and let it remain for about an hour and then strain it and let the patient drink this strained liquid continuously for 5 days.

❑ Take 10 gms, by weight of the root of "Uttarani" (available in ayurvedic shops), and 5 gms. of the powdered seeds of lime (*nimbu*) fruit, mix them well in a little honey and let the patient sip it up little by little.

❑ In the event of a bite by a mad dog, extract about 50 gms, of juice out of the leaves of Indigo plant (Neel), mix it with an equal quantity of cow's milk and let the patient drink it daily for 3 days. The patient should immediately take a course of anti-rabies injections.

REMOVING CIGARETTE ODOUR

❏ To minimise the smell of cigarette smoke in a small room, pour vinegar *(sirka)* in a bowl and keep it in a corner of the room. When the smoke increases, light a candle near the vinegar bowl and feel the difference!

❏ If you light a candle in the room where people are smoking, the non-smokers will not find the cigarette smoke irritating.

❏ To prevent the smell of cigarette from lingering in the room, put half a teaspoon baking powder in the ash tray.

❏ Place a wet sponge in the centre of the room & free the room of tobacco smoke.

RESISTANCE BUILDING OF THE BODY

❏ Papaya is said to have rejuvenating properties & can thus control ageing. Papaya cleanses the body & acts as an excellent tonic & energy giving food.

❏ Oranges or orange juice although acidic in taste has an alkaline reaction in our bodies. After being metabolised it leaves an alkaline residue and thus improves the vital resistance of the body which enables us to fight infections, colds, fevers etc. It also strengthens the bones and increases muscle tone and is good for the nervous system.

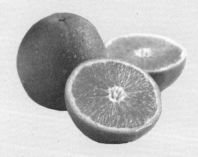

S

SCAR REMOVAL FROM FACE

- Blanch & grind a few almonds to a fine paste with 2 tablespoons milk and one tablespoon each of orange & carrot juice. Apply well on the face and neck. Leave for ½ hour, then wash off.

- Apply one tablespoon finely ground raw papaya on face and neck. Keep for 15-20 minutes and wash off.

- Apply a teaspoon of olive oil mixed with ½ a teaspoon of lemon juice. Leave it for 20-25 minutes & then wash off.

- Apply coconut water (nariyal pani) on the face and leave for 15-20 minutes before washing it off.

- Grind one teaspoon yellow mustard (*peeli rai*) to a paste with 1 tablespoon malai/cream & apply on face and neck. Leave for 15-20 minutes. This also removes itching as well as blemishes from the skin.

- Wash & grind a few fresh mint (*pudina*) leaves to a smooth paste. Apply & leave for ½ hour or apply every night before going to sleep. This helps in getting rid of pimples along with the blemishes.

- Take the pulp of a ripe tomato. Add a few drops of lemon juice & rub on the face and neck. Leave for 20-25 minutes. Wash off.

- If your skin is dry, rub a stick of sandalwood in milk & if skin is oily rub it in rose water (*gulab jal*) and then apply on face. Leave for an hour and then wash with cold water. Very effective during summers.

- For a dry & blemished skin, mix a tablespoon gram flour (*besan*), add a pinch of turmeric (*haldi*), ¼ teaspoon orange peel (*santare ka chilka*) powder, a teaspoon curd (*dahi*) & a teaspoon milk. Apply on face & neck. When skin feels taut, rub it off with finger tips or wash off with tap water.

SEXUAL DEBILITY

What is sexual debility?

Sexual debility is a lack of sexual vitality or inability to perform sex adequately.

Causes...

Over work, stress, under weight and malnourishment.

Symptoms...

Low energy, fatigue, constant tiredness.

Remedy (Nuskhe)...

- ❑ Fry equal quantities of carom (*ajwain*) seeds and kernel of tamarind seeds (*imli ke beej*) in *ghee*. Powder and store in a dry, cool place. Mix 1 teaspoon of this powder in a glass of milk along with 1 tablespoon honey. Drink daily at bedtime.

- ❑ Make *paranthas* of wheat flour by adding ½ cup fenugreek (*methi*) leaves, ½ teaspoon ground almonds, ½ teaspoon poppy seeds (*khuskhus*) and a little ghee. Eat every day for 40 days.

- ❑ Soak 8 to 10 almonds and 1 teaspoon rice overnight. Remove the outer skin, of almonds. Grind both into a fine paste. Mix in some milk and a pinch of turmeric(*haldi*) powder. Boil and drink along with sugar candy (*mishri*) or ordinary sugar to taste.

- ❑ Take 2 teaspoons of amla juice and mix it with two teaspoonfuls each of honey and lemon juice. Add one cup of water and drink on an empty stomach every morning. (*Attention*: The treatment should continue for at least 120 days to achieve expected results).

- ❑ Boil 1 teaspoon ground fenugreek seeds (*methi dana*) in a cup of water & drink.

- ½ teaspoon ginger (*adrak*) juice mixed with honey and a half-boiled egg, taken at night.

- Mix ¼ teaspoon nutmeg (*jaiphal*) powder in a teaspoon honey and take with a half-boiled egg an hour before going to bed.

- Onion seeds (*kalaunji*) dried and powdered, 1 teaspoon eaten 3 times daily along with sugar or honey.

- Boil 1 cup of milk with ½ teaspoon black pepper (*kali mirch*) powder and 6 to 8 crushed almonds. Take at bedtime.

- Grind 2 or 3 teaspoons dried pomegranate seeds (*anaar dana*) and take once or twice along with milk.

- Mix ¼ teaspoon saffron (*kesar*) with milk. Take twice daily.

- Mix sesame seeds (*til*) with jaggery (*gur*) and eat.

SEXUAL VIGOUR & IMPOTENCY

- Mix 2 tablespoon juice of the whitish variety of onions, 1 teaspoon ghee and 1 teaspoon juice of ginger (*adrak*), and about 1½ tablespoon honey. Eat this mixture first thing in the morning for about 4 months or more. This treatment, simple and easy, is a cure for sexual weakness in men and is much better than the fictitious and harmful advertisements in newspapers and magazines.

- Frequent drinking of tender coconut water (*narial paani*) and eating preparations made by using black gram (*urad dal*) will rejuvenate the sexual power of men.

- 2 teaspoons each of roasted and ground fenugreek seeds (*methi daana*) and coriander seeds (*sabut dhania*) mixed with milk or butter and taken every night for a month cures impotency.

- 6 to 8 almonds, crushed & mixed in 1 cup milk along with 1 egg yolk, ½ teaspoon ground sesame seeds (*til*) and 1 teaspoon honey. Take once or twice a day.

SEXUAL WEAKNESS

Remedy (Nuskhe)...

❑ Almonds are basically an energy giving and health building food. It is therefore very beneficial in sexual weakness as its consumption imparts strength. It also gives strength in nervous weakness and helps in sharpening the brain.

❑ As dates are great energy givers they are helpful in cases of sexual weakness. Soak a handful of dates in goat's milk overnight. Remove seed and grind them the next morning. Add a pinch of cardamom (*chhoti ilaichi*) powder and honey to taste. Drink it. This acts as a tonic and is very helpful in overcoming sexual weakness.

❑ Dried figs along with almonds and dried dates (*chhuara*), roasted in butter are said to be beneficial in cases of sexual weakness.

❑ 1 teaspoon of powdered onion seeds (*kalaunji*) eaten 3 times daily along with sugar or honey.

SKIN ALLERGIES

❑ Grind 1 tablespoon poppy seeds (*khus khus*) with 1 teaspoon water. Add 1 teaspoon lemon juice. Apply on the affected areas.

❑ Mix 1 teaspoon lemon juice with sandalwood paste and apply all over.

STOMACH

STOMACH ACHE

- Grind ½ cup mint (*pudina*) with 1" piece of chopped ginger (*adrak*) and juice of ½ lemon in a mixer. Squeeze through a muslin cloth or strain through a fine stainer to get juice. Add ¼ teaspoon black salt (*kala namak*), and take it on an empty stomach.

  When one suffers from gas in the stomach, put a drop of castor oil on the navel, and then press a good pinch of tobacco snuff or asafoetida (*hing*).

- Drink ½ cup warm water with 1 teaspoon ghee and 1 teaspoon sugar for relief from cramps in the stomach.

- A pinch of asafoetida (*hing*) taken along with 1 teaspoon of homemade ghee is an excellent remedy for stomachache.

- Guava (*amrood*) is excellent for indigestion and flatulence (*gas*). People prone to stomach disorders should eat 250 gms, (about 2 small) guavas a day.

- Mix 1 tsp ajwain with ¼ tsp black salt. Chew & eat alone or with warm water if needed.

- Boil 2 tablespoon fennel seeds (*saunf*) in 1 cup water till it is reduce to half. Filter. Take 1 tablespoon every morning and evening for a few days.

- Mix 1 teaspoon mint (*pudina*) juice, 1 teaspoon lemon juice, juice of ¼" piece ginger (*adrak*) and a pinch of black salt (*kala namak*) and drink it.

- Mix a little asafoetida (*hing*) with to make a paste. Apply on and around the navel.

- Drink 1-2 teaspoons brandy with a little warm water. Gives immediate relief from gas.

- Mix carom seeds (*ajwain*) with lemon juice and dry in the sun. Bottle it and have a teaspoon whenever you feel that something is wrong with your stomach (very good for stomach - digestion, gas, indigestion etc.)

- And then there is the age old method of using a hot water bottle and lying down on your stomach to get relief.

STOMACH PAIN AROUND NAVEL

❑ Grind 2 teaspoon each carom seeds (*ajwain*) and dried ginger (*saunth*) into a fine powder. Add a little black salt (*kala namak*). Take 1 teaspoon of this mixture with 1 cup of warm water frequently.

STOMACH, (BURN) BURNING SENSATION

❑ Take 1 teaspoon fenugreek seed (*methi daana*) powder along with milk or buttermilk (*chhachh*) twice daily for a few days.

STOMACH HEAVINESS

❑ Mix ¼ teaspoon each powdered cumin (*jeera*) and black pepper in a glass of buttermilk (*chhachh*). Drink two or three times a day for 2-3 days.

STOMACH ULCERS

Remedy (Nuskhe)...

❑ Drinking coconut water of young green coconut or milk extracted from mature coconut gives quick relief.

STOOLS WITH BLOOD

❑ Take one tablespoon juice of the flower of pomegranate (*anaar*) with sugar candy (*mishri*) twice daily.

STOMACH UPSET (LOOSE MOTIONS)

- ❑ Mashed ripe banana with a little salt, should be taken 2-3 times a day.

- ❑ A teaspoon of date (*khajoor*) paste mixed with a little honey, given three times a day is very effective for regulating the bowels.

- ❑ 5-10 gms of amla seed powder mixed with buttermilk (*chhachh*) should be taken for 1-2 days.

- ❑ Crush 8-10 curry leaves (*curry patta*). Mix with a cup of thin buttermilk (*chhachh*) and have 2-3 times a day.

- ❑ Mix juice of 1 large pomegranate (*anaar*) and 1 glass of sugarcane juice (*ganne ka ras*). Have 4 times a day

- ❑ Fast with only buttermilk, curd, curd and rice, or curd and bananas proves very effective.

- ❑ Avoid raw vegetables and fruits such as orange, mausami, papaya, pineapple and spices.

- ❑ Drink plenty of water to which a teaspoon of sugar and a pinch of salt has been added to guard against dehydration.

- ❑ A strong cup of unsweetened black tea is very effective.

- ❑ A khichdi made with ¼ cup rice and ½ tsp ajwain eaten alone at meal times is very helpful. Roast ajwain in ½ tsp desi ghee. Add rice, pinch of salt and sufficient water. Cook to make a soft khichdi.

- ❑ For children: 1-4 tbsp ripe & sweet apples crushed to a pulp (can be steamed) can be given several times a day.

STAMMERING (HAQLANA)

Remedy (Nuskhe)...

❑ Put 2 black peppercorns (*sabut kali mirch*) in the child's mouth. Suck them for long periods twice a day.

SWEATING EXCESSIVE

Remedy (Nuskhe)...

❑ Mix dry sandalwood powder in rose water (*gulab jal*) (1:1) and apply over parts where sweating is excessive.

SCURVY

What is scurvy?

It is a deficiency disease that results from insufficient intake of vitamin C.

Causes...

Deficiency of vitamin C in the body.

Causes...

- Dark purplish spots on skin, especially legs.
- Spongy gums often leading to tooth loss.
- Bleeding gums.
- Opening of healed scars and separation of knitted bone fractures.

Remedy (Nuskhe)...

❑ Amla is the richest natural source of vitamin C. Consumption of amla in any form will prevent scurvy. When fresh fruit is not available, dried powder can be consumed. As the powder is very sour you can add a little honey to it and have 1-2 teaspoon of amla powder 2-3 times a day with water or milk.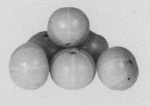

❑ Lemon is also called a poor man's main source of vitamin C as it is very high in vitamin C. It helps cure and prevent scurvy.

❑ Vitamin C deficiency can be overcome by daily consumption of raw mangoes or by consuming *amchoor* - a common spice made from raw mangoes and used for cooking in all Indian households.

TEETHING PROBLEMS IN CHILDREN

❑ Children during teething normally suffer from diarrhoea or dysentery. 1 teaspoon of date paste prepared with honey given 2-3 times a day is very beneficial in overcoming this problem.

THORN, REMOVAL

❑ If a thorn has gone in your or your child's foot and is not coming out, simply mix jaggery (*gur*) and carom seeds (*ajwain*) and tie on it. The thorn will come out on it's own.

THROAT

THROAT, HOARSENESS

❑ Soak 8 to 10 almonds overnight in 1 cup water. After discarding the outer skin, grind the kernels with 8 to 10 black peppers (*sabut kali mirch*) in 1 cup water. Strain it and drink once a day, after adding sugar candy (*mishri*) to taste.

❑ Pour 1 glass boiling water on a mixture of 1 teaspoon each of crushed cinnamon sticks (*dalchini*) and green cardamoms (*chhoti ilaichi*). Keep aside. Filter and use as a gargle when warm.

❑ Boil 2 teaspoons fennel seeds (*saunf*) in barley water and take twice or thrice a day.

❑ Mix seeds of green cardamom (*chhoti ilaichi*) along with 1 tablespoon honey. Eat every day.

THROAT: IRRITATION (*GALE MEIN KHARAASH*)

❏ Gargle 3 times a day with a glass of hot water to which 1 tsp salt has been added.

❏ Boil 1 glass milk with ½ teaspoon turmeric powder *(haldi)* and give 2-3 boils. Strain. Add sugar to taste. Drink at night for 2-3 days before going to bed.

❏ Boil 2 teaspoons carom seeds *(ajwain)* in 2½ cups water for 15 minutes. Strain and add ½ teaspoon salt. Gargle twice a day - early morning and at bed time.

THROAT PAIN, SORE

❏ Crush a few neem leaves with a little water. Strain it. Warm it up. Add a little honey and gargle.

❏ Mix 1 teaspoon lemon juice and 1 tablespoon honey. Swallow tiny amounts slowly 2-3 times a day.

❏ A solution of 2 teaspoons of glycerine and 1 teaspoon of borax powder (*suhaaga*) will give you quick relief from a sore throat. Swirl this mixture in your mouth for a little while with a cotton bud, leave mouth open, bend head in a sink and then let it slide down slowly.

❏ Tender leaves of mango *(aam)* tree help to cure throat ailments and also make the voice sweet. They should be eaten raw daily.

❏ For an effective home remedy for sore throat, cough and cold, boil 1 cup of water with a few mint *(pudina)* leaves till reduced to half the quantity. Strain the boiled water and add 1 teaspoon honey to it. The children will like the sweet taste of honey in it.

❏ Sip or drink slowly 1 cup hot water mixed with juice of ½ lemon *(nimbu)* and 1 teaspoon honey.

❏ Boil 1 glass of milk with a small pinch of ground turmeric *(haldi)*, pepper *(kali mirch)* powder and sugar candy *(mishri)*. Strain it and have it as hot as possible. It relieves throat pain and lung congestion.

❏ Drink tea boiled with ginger *(adrak)* and a few tulsi leaves 2-3 times a day.

❏ Gargle with warm salt water at least twice a day. However do not make gargling sounds as this may aggravate the soreness.

- Pound 2-3 cloves (*laung*), garlic (*lasan*) and add to a cupful of honey. Keep for 1-2 days. Have one teaspoon thrice a day.

- Drink lots of water (10-12 glasses) a day since most throat problems are intensified by dehydration.

- Add 2 tablespoons of fenugreek (*methi*) seeds to 6 cups of water. Heat on low flame for 15-20 minutes. Cool to bearable temperature. Strain and gargle with this, 2-3 times a day.

- Heat a cup of milk till warm. Add 1-2 pinches of turmeric powder (*haldi*), mix well and drink at night.

TOOTHACHE

Remedy (Nuskhe)...

- Pound some asafoetida (*hing*) in a mortar & pestle and add some lemon juice Heat it slightly. Soak a piece of cotton and hold it on the affected area.

- Heat 1 teaspoon coconut oil and fry 3 pieces of cloves (*laung*). Powder. Apply on the affected area.

- Apply nutmeg oil in affected parts.

- Burn the shells of almonds and powder. Use as toothpowder.

- Cotton pad dipped in vanilla essence placed on an aching tooth gives immediate relief.

- Dip a cotton bud in clove oil (*laung ka tel*) and apply on the tooth. Don't apply raw clove oil as this can damage the nerves. Always use a commercial clove oil (*laung ka tel*) meant for this purpose. Powdered black pepper (*kali mirch*) can be mixed with the oil and used.

- For toothache grind 8-10 *tulsi* leaves along with 5-6 peppercorns (*sabut kaali mirch*) and place this paste between the affected teeth or cavity.

- If you have a tooth-ache, boil a few *neem* leaves in two cups water and rinse your mouth a few times with this water. You will get immediate relief from pain.

- A pinch of salt applied to the aching tooth will bring temporary relief.

TYPHOID

What is typhoid?

Also known as "enteric fever". An illness caued by bacteria.

Causes...

Transmitted by ingestion of food or water contaminated by faeces of an infected person.

Symptoms...

In the first week, there is slow rising temperature with headache and cough. Patient feels week, may have diarrhoea or anorexia (loss of appetite).

Remedy (Nuskhe)...

❑ 1 to 2 teaspoon fresh juice of coriander leaves (*hara dhania*) is mixed in 1 cup buttermilk and taken 2-3 times.

❑ Mash a ripe banana along with 1 tablespoon honey and eat twice a day for a few days.

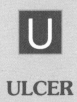

U

ULCER

What is ulcer?

Ulcers are wounds that develop on the mucous membranes. When ulcers affect the gastrointestinal tract, they are called peptic ulcers.

Cause

- Hyperacidity due to heavy meals, highly spiced foods, coffee, alcohol & smoking
- Bacterial infection
- Stress and other psychological factors
- Worsened by certain drugs

Symptoms

Abdominal pain, bloating and abdominal fullness, nausea and vomitting, loss of appetite and weight loss.

Remedy (Nuskhe)...

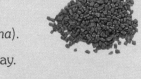

- ❏ Having tea made with fenugreek seeds (*methi daana*).
- ❏ Eating bananas or having banana shake twice a day.
- ❏ A glass of goat's milk taken twice daily.
- ❏ Having milk prepared from blanched almonds.

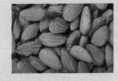

URINATION

Through unination, the body flushes out toxics waste which if allowed to accumlate in the body can lead to major diseses and eventual death. Different kinds of ailments related to urination are listed below alongwith suitable remedies.

URINATION - BURNING

❏ Powder equal quantities of liquorices (*mulethi*) & cumin (*jeera*). Take ¼ teaspoon every day along with 1 teaspoon honey for a month.

❏ Grind 2 or 3 teaspoons dried pomegranate seeds (*anaar daana*) and take once or twice along with milk.

❏ Add 1 to 2 drops of sandalwood oil to milk and take as a night-cap at bedtime.

❏ For burning sensation while passing urine, drink green coconut water (*narial paani*).

URINATION SCANTY

❏ Boil ¼ teaspoon powdered green cardamom (*chhoti ilaichi*) seeds in thin tea water and drink.

❏ Take coconut water, sugar cane juice and barley water often

❏ Take butter milk (*lassi*) with some chopped fresh green coriander (*hara dhania*) with meals.

URINE RETENTION

❏ Soak a little saffron (*kesar*) overnight in ¼ cup water. Next morning drink it with 1 teaspoon honey.

❏ If there is a severe retention of urine, drink 4 tablespoons of castor oil in some warm water for immediate effect (within 15-20 minutes).

- Grind ½ cup cumin seeds (*jeera*) and ½ cup sugar candy *(mishri)* together to a powder. Take 1 teaspoon of this powder three times a day.

- Constantly eating ash gourd (*petha*) in the daily diet will help to prevent urine troubles.

- Eating cucumber (*kheera*) will ward off urine troubles.

- If you put the seeds of wild tulsi in water, a jelly-like liquid is formed. Add a little sugar candy (*mishri*) to this and drink daily for a few days. This will help to release blocked urine.

URINE RETENTION AND ABDOMINAL PAIN

- Add ½ teaspoon camphor (*kapoor*) and 1 tablespoon sandalwood paste to 1 tablespoon warm mustard (*sarson*) oil. Massage gently over the lower abdomen.

- Add 1 to 2 drops of sandalwood oil to milk and take at bedtime.

EXCESSIVE URINATION

- Eat ½ cup roasted gram (*bhune channe*) and then eat a small piece of jaggery (*gur*) after that, for about 10 days.

- Grapes and spinach (*paalak ki subzi*) are good in controlling excessive urination.

- A jaggery and sesame seeds laddu (*gur aur til ka laddu*), taken every morning and evening during winters is very helpful. Have it for 4-5 days.

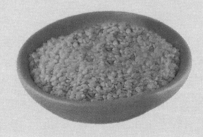

VARICOSE VEINS

❑ Consumption of jamuns proves specially beneficial as they contain antioxidants-anthocyanin and ronthocyanidin, which help to strengthen and tone the venous walls so that they do not swell and bleed.

VERTIGO

What is vertigo?

Dizziness or "spinning" sensation while the body is stationary.

Causes...

Usually associated with a problem in the inner-ear balance mechanism in the brain, or the nerve connections between these two organs.

Symptoms...

Can cause nausea and vomitting, or if severe, may give rise to difficulty in standing or walking.

Remedy (Nuskhe)...

❑ Soak 1 teaspoon each of dried amla powder and coriander seeds (*sabut dhania*) in water overnight. Strain and drink next morning. To improve the flavour, sugar can be added. Repeat for a few days.

- Heat 2 tablespoon sesame oil (*til ka tel*). Mix in ½ teaspoon each of finely powdered cardamom (*chhoti ilaichi*) and cinnamon (*dalchini*). Apply on head.

- Mix 7 to 8 almonds with 7 to 8 kernels of pumpkin (*kaddu*) seeds, 1 teaspoon poppy seeds (*khus khus*) and 3 tablespoons wheat. Soak in water overnight. Next morning, remove the outer skin of the almonds and grind together into a fine paste. Heat separately 2 teaspoons ghee and fry ½ teaspoon cloves (*laung*). Add the paste to it along with some milk and boil the whole mixture. Sweeten with sugar and drink every day for a few days.

VIGOUR

- Walnuts impart vigour and remove impotency.

VOMITTING AND NAUSEA

Remedy (Nuskhe)...

- Licking the powder of fried cloves (*laung*) mixed with honey controls vomitting.

- Sucking a piece of ice also controls vomitting.

- Mix 2-3 teaspoon of curry leaves (*curry patta*) juice with a teaspoon of lemon juice (can add little sugar if needed). Drinking this will control morning sickness, nausea and vomitting.

- Crush 2-3 cloves of garlic (*lasan*) and boil with ¾ cup of water or milk. Boil till half the amount remains and then drink. It takes care of all digestive disorders.

- Mix ½ teaspoon of fresh ginger (*adrak*) juice with 1 teaspoon each of freshlime, mint (*pudina*) juice and 1 tablespoon of honey and drink.

- Slice a ripe banana. Sprinkle some powdered sugar and freshly ground cardamoms (*chhoti ilaichi*) on top. Eat 1-2 times a day.

- Eat ½ teaspoon ground cumin seeds (*jeera*).

- Ginger (*adrak*) tea or sucking sliced ginger helps.

- Powdered cinnamon (*dalchini*) and sliced ginger (*adrak*) work by interrupting nausea signals sent from the stomach to the brain. If you are a herbal tea drinker, simply sprinkle powdered cinnamon on the tea and drink. To make ginger tea, simmer a few slices of ginger in hot tea water.

- Mix ½ teaspoon lemon juice with ½ teaspoon honey and lick 2-3 times a day. This remedy is very helpful in checking and controlling vomitting.

- Crush 2 cloves *(laung)* and boil in ½ cup water. When half the water remains, strain and add sugar candy *(mishri)* to taste. Have it 4 times a day, ¼ cup each time and lie down on the side after drinking this.

VOMITTING DUE TO INDIGESTION

- Frequent intake of lemon juice is a good remedy.

WARTS

Remedy (Nuskhe)...

❑ Mash the garlic (*lasan*) cloves and apply externally.

❑ Apply the milky juice exuding from the stems of figs (*anjeer*) and leaves on the affected areas.

❑ Place some chopped onions in a dish, cover with salt and leave overnight. Twice a day apply the resulting juice to the warts until they disappear.

❑ Another alternative is fresh pineapple juice or slices. Since pineapple contains an enzyme that breaks down warts, it is very effective in removing warts without leaving behind any marks. Apply some to the wart several times a day until it has gone.

WEIGHT GAIN

❑ Mango is a very nourishing fruit. It is rich in sugar and hence the consumption of mangoes is beneficial for people who are underweight. In fact a combination of mango and milk taken 3-4 times a day is highly recommended for weight gain. Milk has no sugar and mango has no protein, whereas mango is rich in sugar and milk in protein. Therefore they compliment each other very well.

WEIGHT REDUCTION

❑ Watermelon (tarbooz) is an ideal fruit for people wanting to lose weight. It contains a large amount of water and is very low in its calorie content. Consuming watermelon once or twice a day fills you up and although your stomach is full you have consumed very few calories and hence it aids in weight reduction.

WHEAT GRASS THERAPY

Wheat grass juice cures ailments ranging from common cold to many other chronic diseases. It contains all the minerals essential for our body. The most vital ingredient being  chlorophyll. It is similar to haemoglobin in our blood & hence dieticians call it green blood. It purifies blood, boosts up the functioning of heart, lungs & kidneys.

This therapy is said to be effective in all diseases of the body like high blood pressure, anaemia, acidity, nausea, worms, diabetes, pimples, boils, bronchitis, common cold, asthma, ulcers, insomnia, headache, piles, deficiency of vitamin A, swelling & pain in joints etc.

Wheat grass juice should be taken daily, early in the morning for at least 21 days continuously. Do not consume anything for 30-40 minutes after drinking the juice. The *Dosage of juice* for various illnesses is given below:

1. Ordinary illness or common ailment - 100 ml. (about ½ tea cup) per day.
2. For serious & chronic diseases - Start with 50 ml (about ¼ tea cup) per day & gradually increase the dosage to 200-250 ml (1 tea cup) per day.

It is advisable to take 50 ml of the juice every day in order to maintain proper health for any normal person.

How to get Wheat Grass Juice

Wheat grass are the young shoots of wheat. You can grow them in small pots in your house. Use seven pots & sow wheat in one pot every day. When the shoots are 4-5 inches long in the first pot, cut them. Wash and grind along with water in the mixer. Sieve & drink first thing in the morning. By using 7 pots you ensure a fresh pot full of wheat grass for 7 days. However, if you keep repeating the cycle you get an endless supply of fresh wheat grass for your therapy.

WATER THERAPY

Several chronic diseases for which no cure has been found can be cured by a simple method called water therapy. Several diseases such as headaches, hypertension, obesity, diabetes, arthritis, sinusitis, bronchitis, bronchial asthma, acidity, gastritis, constipation, irregular mensuration etc. are cured by this therapy. Though it sounds incredible, it has been proved & is recommended by several doctors. However, individual results may vary.

How to Practice

The method of practising water therapy is simple, easy & inexpensive. Early in the morning before attending to any of the morning chores (as soon as you wake up), drink 5 glasses of water (1.25 litres) at a stretch. If you cannot drink them at a stretch, give a small break & then complete the drinking of the water. However do not do any exercise before you finish drinking the rest of the water. For the next 45 minutes to 1 hour, do not consume anything. During the first few days of therapy, one may pass urine very frequently and some may even have loose motions/stools. But within a few days everything becomes normal and a relief from the symptoms of the disease will be seen. While practising water therapy, always drink water 2 hours after meals & not before that.

Using Water for Curing Diseases

❑ Sipping water slowly: Hot water when sipped slowly, cleans the stomach, relieves heartburn, acute indigestion, vomitting and cramps in the abdomen.

   Caution! Hot water is not recommended for those who suffer from ulcers in the abdomen.

❑ Water and high B.P: Water taken sufficiently, can also delay the onset of high blood pressure. Drinking water, kept in a copper vessel overnight, drunk the next day is very helpful in bringing down the blood pressure.

- Water and bladder infection: Bladder infection also benefits from forced drinking. This has been proved medically. The water flushes out bacteria and inflammatory debris from the bladder.

- Hot water bath is ideal for Arthritis: Hot water has curative properties.

Water as Sedative - Cure for Sleeplessness

There is nothing in the world better for insomnia than a hot bath. A 15 minutes warm bath before going to bed will cure sleeplessness. It relaxes the blood vessels of the skin. It also soothes the nerve endings, helping to calm you down if you're feeling nervous. In fact, before the advent of tranquillizing drugs, natural baths were used with great success in calming agitated mental patients.

Always Remember...

Drink 8 to 10 glasses of water per day. Do not drink water only when you feel thirsty. Research has proved that when you feel thirsty, the thirst damages your body. Therefore, do not wait for a glass of water till you are thirsty. Keep taking water off and on to prevent the damage from lack of water consumption. Do not depend upon your thirst mechanism to drink water.

TULSI - THE WONDER HERB

This holy plant possesses multiple curative properties. From ancient times, our ancestors believed in the spiritual and healing properties of this plant. Science has proved that regular consumption of Tulsi for 3 months can cure diseases like frequent occurence of Cough & Cold, Headache, Eyestrain, Old age weakness, Loose motions, High and Low blood pressure, Heart troubles, Obesity, Acidity, Constipation, Kidney troubles, Stones & Gout pains.

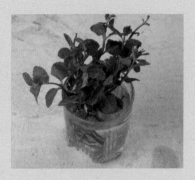

It strengthens the body to fight diseases resulting from deficiency of Vitamin A and Vitamin C. Consumption of Tulsi can also cure body wrinkles, diseases related to women, skin problems and fever. This can also benefit people suffering from Cancer.

Preparing Tulsi Medicine

Take 30-35 clean Tulsi leaves and crush to a paste. Mix 1-2 tablespoons of sweet curd (dahi) with it. If curd does not suit you mix the tulsi paste with 1-2 teaspoons of honey. Take this mixture (medicine) on an empty stomach in the mornings for 3 months. Breakfast can be taken after 1 hour. The medicine should be taken only once a day for 3 months but in the case of cancer and other painful, chronic diseases it can be taken 2-3 times a day.

Caution! Curd (*dahi*) used should not be sour.

In the case of children ¼ teaspoon of Tulsi paste should be mixed with a little honey and not with curd. Do not mix the paste with milk for children.

VISUALISATION

(MIND OVER BODY)

Positive thinking can be a powerful tool in combating a wide number of ailments or illnesses. Using power of your will to overcome ill-health is not new—it's been used throughout centuries. We can see cases in our daily life, who are surviving only by their strong will power, contrary to doctors verdict. We take it as a miracle.

The scientists are now accepting this principle. Instead of calling 'Mind Power', they call it Visualization. It has been proved through medical research, to be an extremely powerful weapon for curing diseases.

Decide exactly what it is that you want your visualizing to accomplish. This could be something of short term—like getting rid of a headache–or more long-term such as making your digestive system work correctly.

THE MIRACLE CHEMICAL

ENDORPHIN is a chemical manufactured in the brain which prevents, treats and may cure any disease, including cancer and AIDS, without side effects. It eliminates all the pains.

The scientists found out that Endorphin not only makes a human happy, but it can also makes human body healthier through production of Lymphocytes, i.e., one of many white blood cells. These are defence cells that fight many diseases and can be referred to as soldiers, policemen and doctors of our body.

In AIDS patients these white blood cells decrease, thus diminishing the immunity of the patient. We can produce more endorphins by the following methods:

Humour Thyselves

Research showed that laugh and smile produces Rs.100,000 worth of endorphins – a finding that justifies the Oriental teachings that a smile brings wealth and happiness. Start using these 3 tips and produce good quantity of this wonderful and miraculous chemical and make yourself happy and healthy.

❑ Use the mantra 'It does not matter' frequently.

❑ Laugh consciously at least once a day.

❑ Be over a situation rather than be in it.

Prayer and Meditation

If you meditate with happiness and a smiling face, you can feel the endorphins flow all through you and a glow comes to your face. This may explain how some prayer leads to miraculous disappearance of diseases.

INDEX

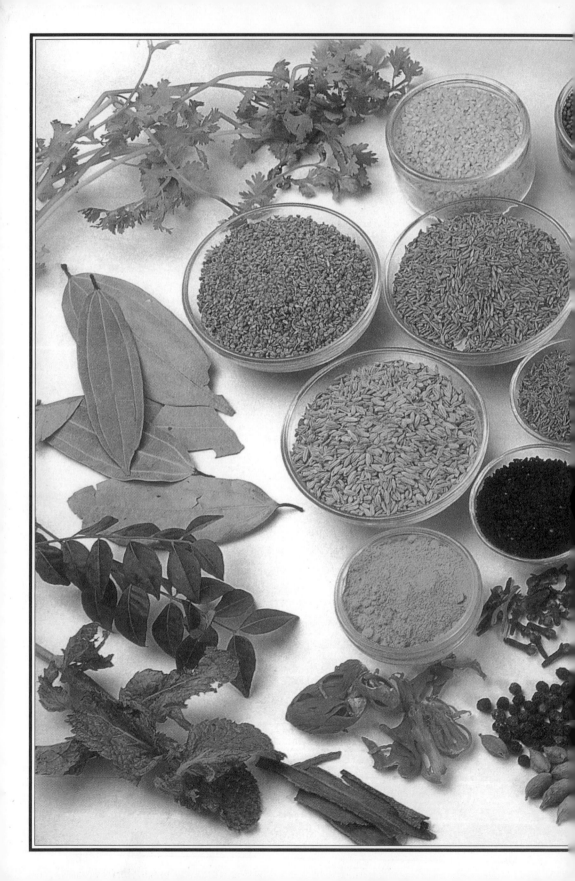